55 00
05

A Colour Atlas of

SURGICAL MANAGEMENT OF VENOUS DISEASE

C. VAUGHAN RUCKLEY
MB; ChM; FRCSE
Consultant Surgeon, Vascular Surgery Unit
Royal Infirmary and part-time Senior Lecturer
University Department
of Clinical Surgery, Edinburgh

Photography by:
Henry J Philip and
James E McGowan
Department of Medical Photography,
Royal Infirmary, Edinburgh

Wolfe Medical Publications Ltd

Copyright © C. Vaughan Ruckley, 1988
Published by Wolfe Medical Publications Ltd, 1988
Printed by W.S. Cowell Ltd., Ipswich, United Kingdom
ISBN 0 7234 0898 X

For a full list of other titles published by
Wolfe Medical Publications Ltd, please write
to the publishers at Brook House, 2-16 Torrington
Place, London WC1E 7LT, England.

A CIP catalogue record for this book is available from the
British Library, 2 Sheraton Street, London W1A 6JZ.

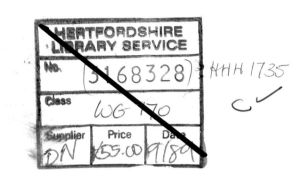
TITLES OF RELATED INTEREST

SURGERY FOR VARICOSE VEINS
C. Vaughan Ruckley *0 7234 1001 1*

PERIPHERAL VASCULAR DISEASES
William F. Walker *0 7234 0738 X*

VASCULAR SURGERY
John S. P. Lumley *0 7234 9033 1*

REDUCING OPERATIONS FOR LYMPHOEDEMA OF LOWER LIMB
M. L. Browse *0 7234 1043 7*

EXTRACRANIAL/INTRACRANIAL ANASTOMOSIS
John S. P. Lumley *0 7234 1012 7*

EXTRA-ANATOMIC BYPASS FOR LOWER LIMB VASCULAR DISEASE
John Chamberlain *0 7234 1015 1*

VISCERAL ARTERY RECONSTRUCTION
Adrian Marston *0 7234 1036 4*

OPERATIONS ON THE INTERNAL CAROTID ARTERY
H. H. G. Eastcott *0 7234 1023 2*

Contents

Preface

The surgery of venous disease constitutes a large part of the work of the general surgeon. Although frequently entrusted to junior and inexperienced hands it is often difficult surgery or, to be more precise, it is difficult to carry out successfully. For supporting evidence one needs to look no further than the very great frequency with which varicose veins and varicose ulcers recur.

This book is concerned mainly with the management of common venous disorders, concentrating on those procedures that are relevant to general and vascular surgical practice everywhere. It is aimed at the practising surgeon, in particular the surgical trainee, but it has been set out in a way which I hope will offer something of interest to undergraduates and to all those medical and nursing staff concerned with the care of patients with venous disorders in operating theatres, clinics and wards.

I have not attempted to cover in detail every aspect of venous surgery. For example, the transplantation and repair of vein valves are mentioned only briefly because these techniques, in my view, remain to be validated as safe and worthwhile for general adoption.

Acknowledgements

The following people generously provided illustrations and/or advice: Dr Paul Allan, Dr Doris Redhead, Dr Paul Buxton, Mr Simon Darke, Mr Arthur Gardner, Dr Terence Ryan and Mr Anthony Watson. My colleagues in the Lothian and Forth Valley Leg Ulcer Study, Mr Michael Callam, Mrs Jaqueline Dale and Mr Douglas Harper, kindly gave permission for me to include material from that project. Three companies also assisted with material for illustrations: W L Gore & Associates (UK), William Cook Europe, and Acuscan. Mr Henry Philip and Mr James McGowan showed great skill and patience in obtaining the photographs in the operating theatre, clinics and studio. My wife, Anne, spent many hours helping me to review the text and illustrations. My most grateful thanks to all.

1 Anatomy

In the dissecting room scant attention is paid to the superficial veins and often the deep veins are not clearly visible, attention being concentrated on the arterial supply to organs and structures. And yet in few areas of surgery is an intimate knowledge of anatomy so closely linked to successful treatment. This particularly applies to an awareness of the many variations to which the venous system is peculiarly liable.

This section illustrates areas which are important either because they relate to venous haemodynamics (for example, the pumps of foot and calf, valves, the deep fascia) or because they are the focal points of common operations (for example, the saphenofemoral and saphenopopliteal junctions, perforators). For a full account of venous anatomy the reader should consult a reference text[1].

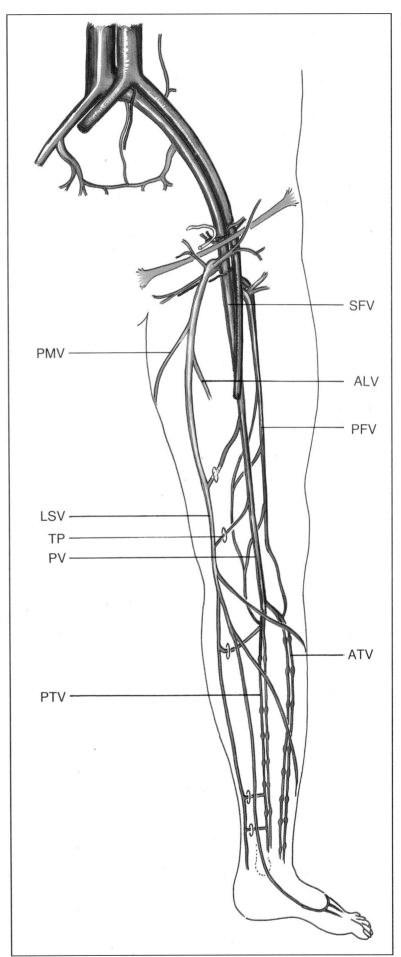

1a Veins of the lower limb.

SFV – superficial femoral vein
ALV – anterolateral vein
PMV – posteromedial vein
PFV – profunda femoris vein
LSV – long saphenous vein
TP – thigh perforator vein
PV – popliteal vein
ATV – anterior tibial vein
PTV – posterior tibial vein

Veins of the lower limb

The venous foot pump

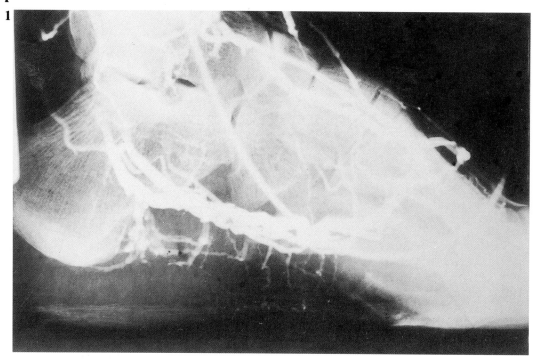

1 Although foot volumentry (page 23) has gained an established place in the vascular laboratory, the venous return from the foot has not been well understood until recently. Gardner and Fox have demonstrated that the capacious, plexiform medial plantar veins, in contrast to the veins of the calf pump, are emptied by weight bearing rather than by muscle contraction[2].

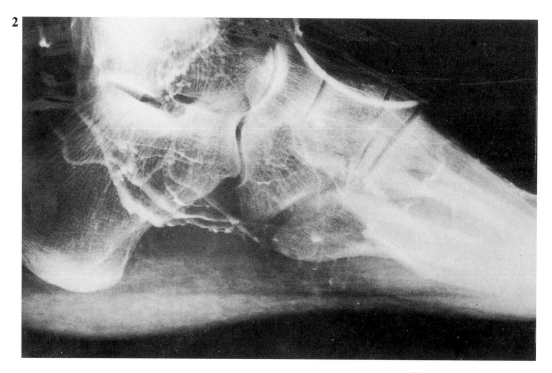

2 External compression of the sole, as in the transfer of weight, results in a pulse which can be demonstrated readily by Doppler ultrasound in the popliteal and femoral veins.

The calf muscle pump

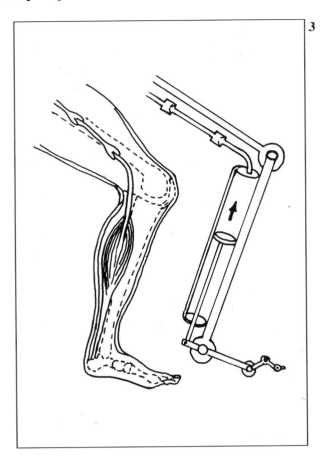

3

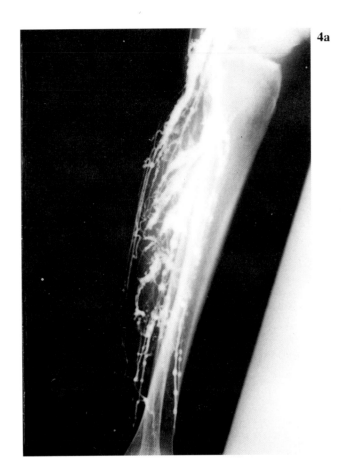

4a

3 During normal walking the systolic contractions of the soleus and gastrocnemius muscles generate pressures. These are greater than 100 mmHg within the posterior compartment. Thus the deep veins and, in particular, the intramuscular veins are evacuated. Normally the superficial veins are protected from this pressure by valves in the perforating veins.

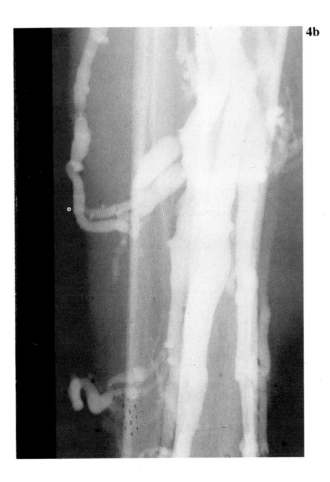

4b

4a This lateral view of an ascending phlebogram shows the paired sinusoidal intramuscular veins of the calf muscle pump. The somewhat irregular appearance of the sinusoids is due to previous deep vein thrombosis (DVT).

4b In this anteroposterior view of an ascending phlebogram the deep veins are dilated and lack the beaded appearance of normal calf valve sinuses, which suggests the presence of deep vein incompetence. The intramuscular veins connect with a varicose superficial vein via a perforator.

The superficial veins

The superficial veins lie in three strata[3]. The long and the short saphenous veins for most of their courses are applied closely to the deep fascia accompanied respectively by the saphenar and sural nerves. The second layer of veins, lying between the deep fascia and the membranous layer of the superficial fascia, consists of the main tributaries of the saphenous veins, such as the anterolateral and posteromedial veins of the thigh and the arch veins of the calf. The third layer comprises veins lying between the skin and the membranous layer of the superficial fascia. They are thin-walled, poorly supported, distend readily and become tortuous.

The long saphenous vein (LSV)

5 The long (*syn*. great, internal) saphenous vein arises from the medial end of the dorsal venous arch of the foot. It is relatively constant in position where it crosses the medial malleolus obliquely to ascend posteromedially in the calf and thigh. It lies on the deep fascia except at the level of the knee joint where it is more superficial, a point of importance when it is being dissected out for arterial bypass. Its principal tributaries are the anterior and posterior arch veins of the calf which join it just below the knee and which connect it with perforating veins and the anterolateral and posteromedial veins of the thigh which join it between 5 cm and 15 cm below the saphenofemoral junction. The latter may form a connection with the short saphenous vein (SSV); this is a substantial channel in those cases where the short saphenous vein fails to join the popliteal vein.

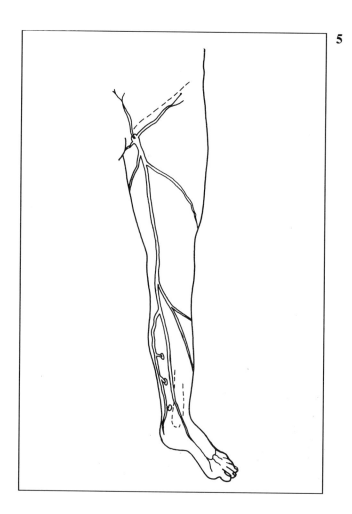

The saphenofemoral junction

6 Three centimetres below and lateral to the pubic tubercle the long saphenous vein turns inwards piercing the cribiform fascia to pass through the foramen ovale, where it joins the common femoral vein. Typically the long saphenous vein receives **three** tributaries as it turns through the foramen ovale: the **superficial external pudendal**, the **superficial inferior epigastric** and the **superficial circumflex iliac veins**. The deep external pudendal vein joins the medial side of the common femoral vein at the level of the saphenofemoral junction. Occasionally it joins the long saphenous vein. The deep external pudendal artery crosses the common femoral vein immediately below the saphenofemoral junction.

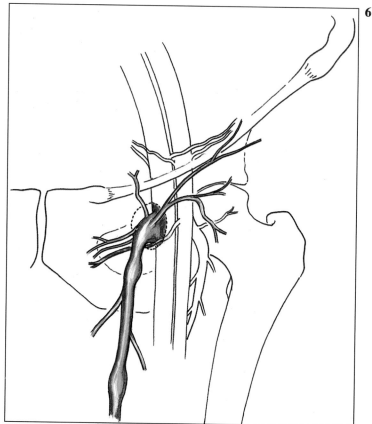

Variations in the long saphenous vein

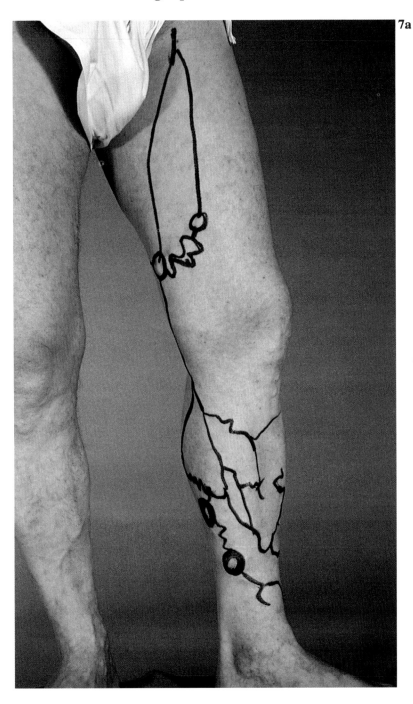

7a

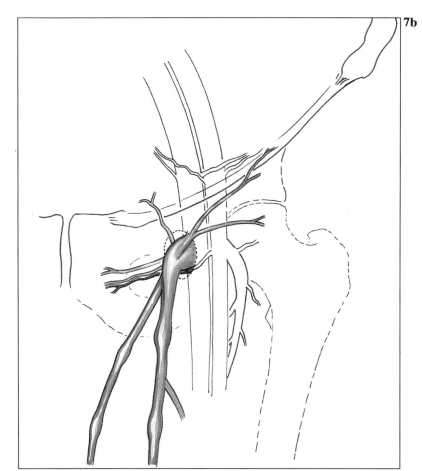

7b

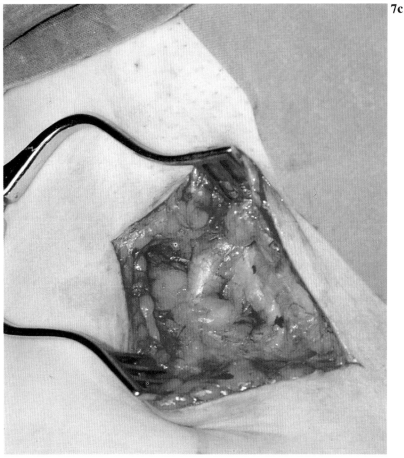

7c

7a Variations in anatomy in the femoral region are frequent. They are an important cause of failure of varicose vein surgery[4]. In this example a large posteromedial tributary joins the saphenous vein close to the junction. Unless the area is properly dissected out, the tributary may be ligated in mistake for the saphenous vein which is thus left intact. An example seen at operation is shown on page 43.

7b In this patient with primary varicose veins, physical examination revealed two large trunks converging on the saphenofemoral junction.

7c Incision over the saphenofemoral junction confirmed that instead of a single long saphenous vein, there were two large trunks. Further dissection in this case is shown on page 43.

8 Here the anterolateral tributary joins the superficial circumflex iliac vein instead of the saphenous vein directly. If the tributaries are simply ligated close to the saphenous vein, recurrence will inevitably follow. The tributaries should be dissected several centimetres out from the junction and the confluent veins should be ligated separately.

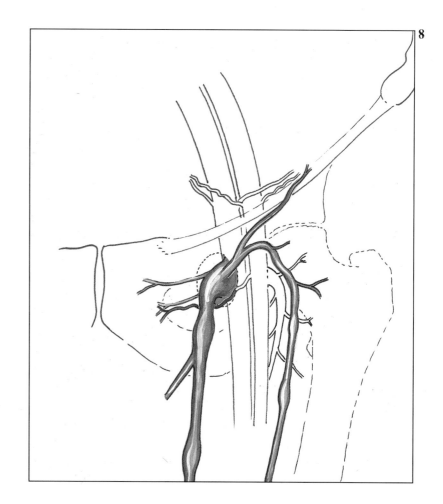

9 An operative dissection showing this type of abnormality.

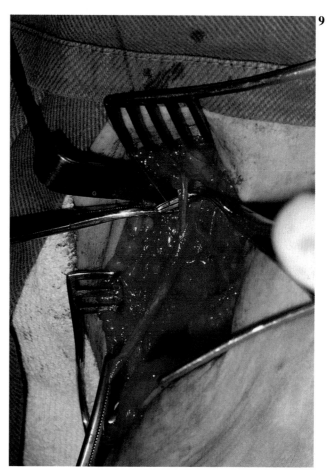

The short saphenous vein (SSV)

The short (*syn.* lesser, external) saphenous vein arises on the lateral side of the foot and in about two-thirds of individuals it terminates in the popliteal fossa. It passes with the sural nerve below and then behind the lateral malleous. It is applied to the deep fascia in the lower third of the calf where it runs along the lateral border of the tendo calcaneus and then up the median line of the calf. It enters a fascial tunnel in the gastrocnemius sheath in the middle third of the calf; in the upper third it penetrates the deep fascia to enter the popliteal space where it passes forward either medial or lateral to the medial popliteal nerve.

The saphenopopliteal junction

10 The short saphenous vein usually enters the popliteal space 1-2 cm below the transverse skin crease. This point is quite variable as is the point of entry into the popliteal vein, which is generally 2-3 cm proximal to the transverse crease. In about a third of cases it is several centimetres higher and in about 15 per cent it joins the deep veins or the long saphenous vein in the upper third of the calf. Before it terminates it gives off a branch which ascends medially to join the long saphenous and it receives a descending median thigh vein, a remnant of the postaxial vein. It may also be joined by a gastrocnemius vein before it joins the popliteal vein. In the lower third of the calf the short saphenous is joined by a lateral ankle perforating vein which connects it with the peroneal vein. There is also commonly a perforator which connects with the intramuscular veins at about mid calf.

There is often sacculation of the proximal end of the short saphenous vein. A rare anomaly is termination of the short saphenous vein in phlebectasia of the vasa vasorum of the sciatic nerve or one of its divisions [5].

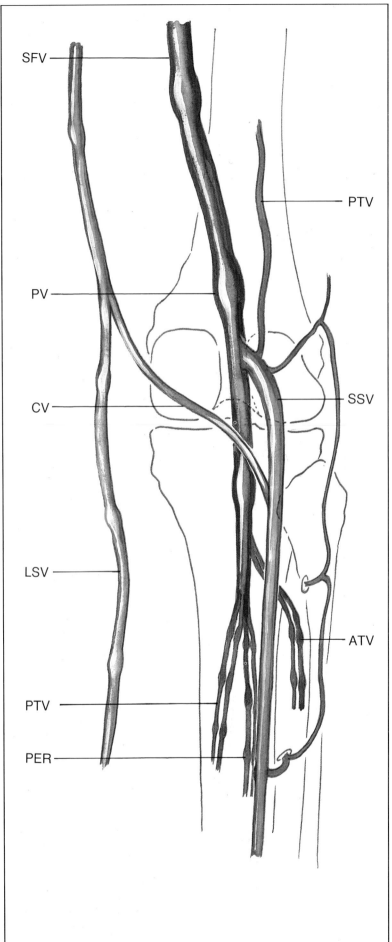

SFV – superficial femoral vein
PTV – posterior thigh vein
PV – popliteal vein
CV – connecting vein between short saphenous and long saphenous veins
SSV – short saphenous vein
LSV – long saphenous vein
ATV – anterior tibial vein
PTV – posterior tibial vein
PER – peroneal vein

Deep veins

11 The deep veins are paired as they accompany the tibial and peroneal arteries. The saccular intramuscular veins, within the muscle belly of soleus are also paired. They drain principally into the posterior tibial veins. Those within the gastrocnemius enter the popliteal vein in the popliteal fossa. The popliteal and femoral veins are often also paired. There is anastomosis between the veins of the popliteal fossa and the profunda femoris system which ensures that thrombosis of the femoral vein in the thigh does not *per se* give rise to obstructive symptoms[6]. The medullary cavities of the long bones also connect liberally with the deep veins, a fact formerly made use of frequently in intraosseous phlebography.

In this patient there is thrombus in the peroneal veins extending into the popliteal veins.

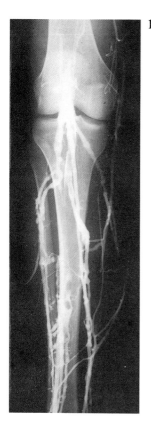

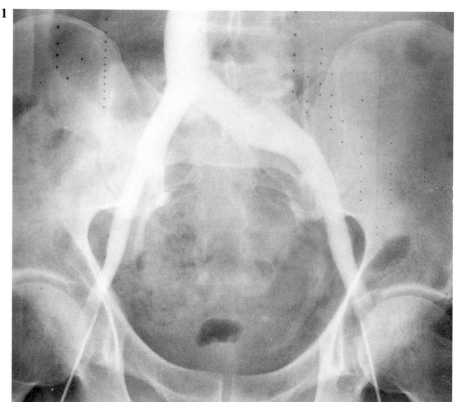

Pelvic veins

12 The right common iliac vein and the cava are almost in line. The left common iliac vein joins at more of an angle and is compressed by the overlying right common iliac artery. In one in five individuals there is a web or band at the mouth of the left common iliac vein. The adoption of the erect posture has rendered the great veins of the lower abdomen and pelvis susceptible to pressure by contiguous organs, notably the left colon and the pregnant uterus. These features are assumed to account for the greater frequency of venous thrombosis in the left leg and the greater frequency in women.

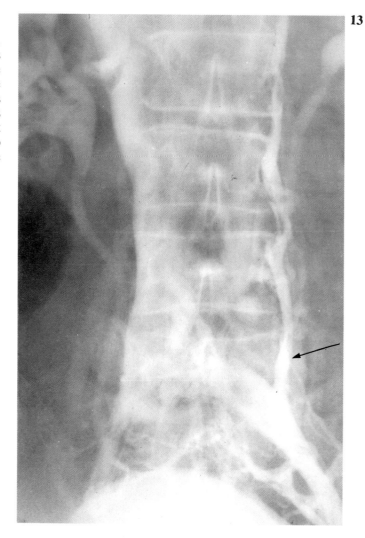

13 The iliolumbar vein (arrowed) is sometimes quite large. This is one of the reasons why venous thrombectomy is best performed under fluoroscopic control. A thrombectomy catheter passed upwards from the left groin readily enters this vein which may then rupture when the balloon is inflated.

14 There are numerous connections between the two iliac systems. These are mainly across the floor of the pelvis via the internal iliacs. Therefore, an occlusion confined to a common iliac vein will impede the venous return from the leg very little but if the internal iliac vein is also obstructed, the symptoms are likely to be severe.

This patient had an occlusion of the inferior vena cava which has caused filling of the very numerous collateral channels.

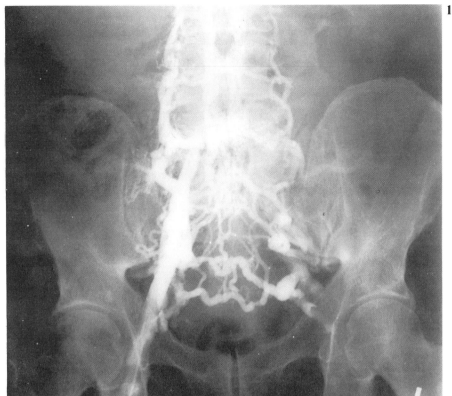

Deep fascia

15 The deep fascia which separates the deep and superficial systems forms a continuous cylinder fused at the top of the thigh with the ligaments and periosteum of the pelvis, at the knee with the capsule of the knee joint and at the ankle with the retinacular ligaments. It is traversed by the terminal parts of the saphenous veins and by a number of perforating or communicating veins accompanied by small arteries. Here the deep fascia has been lifted up to display the underlying muscle and a perforating vein.

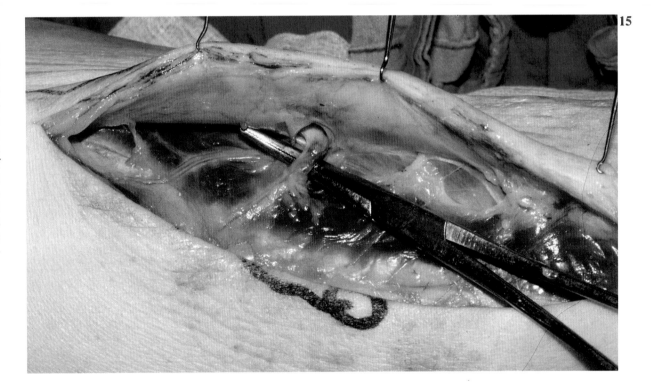

Perforating veins

16 In the calf the perforating veins seldom pass directly from the main saphenous trunks to the deep veins. They pass from tributaries such as the posterior arch vein of the calf. For this reason there appears to be no advantage in stripping the long saphenous vein in the calf when dealing with perforator incompetence.

The large perforators such as those in the gaiter area at the medial border of soleus and the mid-Hunter perforator in the lower thigh pass directly to the main subjacent deep veins, that is the paired tibial veins and the femoral veins respectively. Higher in the calf a number of small perforators, usually of little surgical importance, connect with intramuscular veins.

17 Thigh perforators in contrast usually pass direct from the saphenous stem [7].

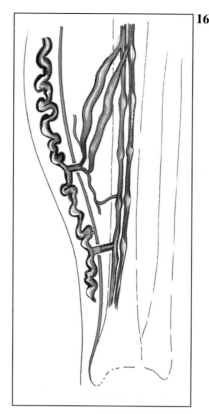

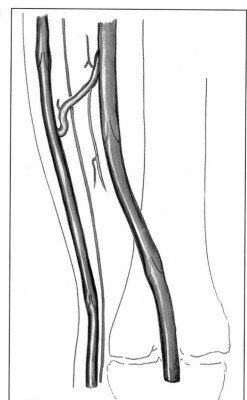

Valves

18 Valves are liberally distributed throughout the deep and superficial systems up to the level of the groin. The valves are more frequent in the more peripheral veins. They are delicate translucent bicuspid structures formed of endothelial folds. Of particular strategic importance are the valves at the points of connection between the deep and superficial systems: the saphenofemoral junction, the saphenopopliteal junction and the perforating veins.

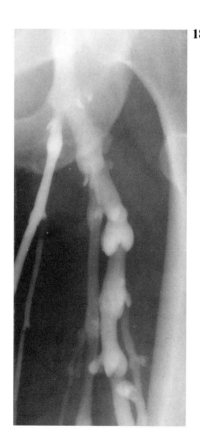

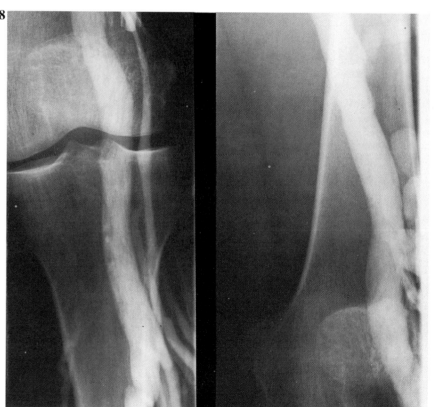

19 When the valves are defective, the deep veins take on a characteristically featureless 'canal-like' appearance on phlebography (see also Fig. **4b**).

Veins of the upper limb

The venous drainage comprises a deep and a superficial system both of which drain into a common trunk, the axillary vein.

20 The deep veins are paired, accompanying the arteries. They possess valves. The axillary vein begins as a continuation of the basilic vein opposite the lower border of the teres major muscle and becomes the subclavian vein at the outer border of the first rib. With the exception of the acromiothoracic vein which joins the cephalic, its tributaries correspond to the branches of the axillary artery. It also receives the cephalic vein at the upper border of the pectoralis minor muscle.

The two largest superficial veins of the upper limb are the cephalic and the basilic which derive from the medial and lateral sides respectively of the dorsal network of the hand. The cephalic ascends on the lateral border of the biceps, then in the deltopectoral groove to the infraclavicular fossa where it turns medially to pierce the clavipectoral fascia and enter the axillary vein. It is connected to the basilic vein at the elbow,

The basilic vein ascends along the ulnar border at the back of the forearm and then passes forwards to ascend at the medial border of the biceps. At about the middle of the arm it pierces the deep fascia and ascends on the medial side of the brachial artery to become the axillary vein.

The subclavian vein begins at the outer border of the first rib. Laterally, as it enters the costoclavicular space, it rests on the first rib and pleura and lies behind the subclavian muscle, the costocoracoid ligament (a condensation of the clavipectoral fascia) and the medial part of the clavicle. The subclavian vein crosses the scalenus anterior muscle which separates it from the second part of the subclavian artery. At the medial border of the scalenus anterior it joins the internal jugular vein to become the brachiocephalic vein behind the medial end of the clavicle.

Each subclavian vein has a bicuspid valve immediately lateral to the junction with the internal jugular. The brachiocephalic veins do not contain valves.

In certain positions of the arm and shoulder the costoclavicular space is narrowed by a scissor-like action of first rib and clavicle, which in some individuals is sufficient to obstruct the vein. These positions are first the 'military' position with the shoulders braced back and downward traction on the arms. The second is full abduction plus external rotation at the shoulder.

Although in some individuals a narrow costoclavicular gap is sufficient to cause thoracic outlet obstruction, usually it is an anatomical abnormality which is responsible, the best known being cervical rib. In fact abnormal fibromuscular bands are a commoner cause of outlet obstruction than cervical rib. These have been classified into ten varieties by Roos [8].

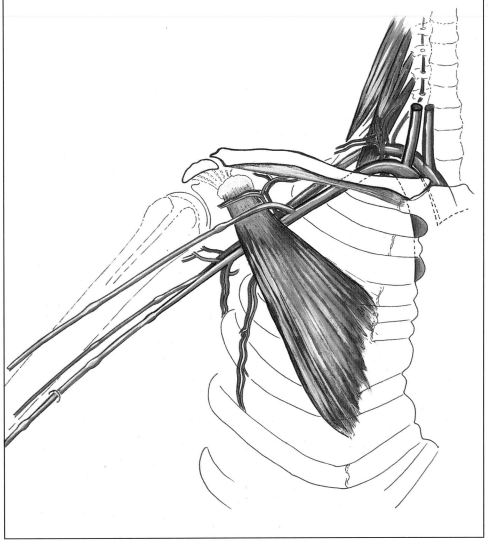

20

2 Assessment

This chapter is concerned mainly with the assessment of patients with varicose veins and other forms of chronic venous disease. The section on phlebography also includes the investigation of patients with deep venous thrombosis and pulmonary embolism, the treatment of which is discussed in Chapter 11.

History

Uncomplicated varicose veins give rise to relatively few symptoms. Dilated segments often feel tender and ache on standing. The legs may feel tired and heavy and swelling may be noticed towards the end of the day. These symptoms are aggravated by hormonal changes, especially around the menopause. Pain from osteoarthritis, sciatic root compression and arterial insuffucuency is often mistaken for varicose veins. If the symptoms are not alleviated by the wearing of graduated compression stockings, they are unlikely to be caused by the veins and will not be relieved by sclerotherapy or surgery.

Conversely it is wrong to assume, because there are no visible varices, that posture-related symptoms are not venous in origin. For example, discomfort in the calf on prolonged standing, usually in female patients, can be shown to be related to distension of gastrocnemius veins, best seen on a lateral view ascending phlebogram.

Some patients are anxious that they may develop varicose ulcers, while others are more concerned about the immediate unsightliness of the varices. The latter group should be warned that surgery leaves scars, however small, that sclerotherapy often leaves pigmentation and that varices have a natural tendency to recur after treatment.

Patients with primary varicose veins will usually have a FAMILY HISTORY of varicose disease. Careful enquiry should be made as to previous PHLEBITIS, DVT or PULMONARY EMBOLISM. Often a DVT will not have been recognised as such, but closer questioning will elicit a history of leg-swelling after trauma, particularly lower limb fractures, in the puerperium or in the postoperative period. If SWELLING is a prominent symptom, the deep veins are likely to be incompetent or occluded. Venous CLAUDICATION, especially if the symptoms are aggravated by elastic compression, suggests occlusion of the iliofemoral segment with inadequate collateral channels.

A history of DIABETES or symptoms of ARTERIAL INSUFFICIENCY whether cardiac, cerebral or peripheral should alert one to the potential dangers of elastic compression. Examples of tissue damage caused by elastic stockings and by bandages are shown on pages 97 and 117.

A careful note should be made of PREVIOUS TREATMENTS either of veins or of skin conditions. A history of ALLERGIC REACTIONS is important, both in the patient who requires a phlebogram and where dressings are needed for the skin complications of chronic venous insufficiency (see Chapter 14).

Physical examination

1 The patient is examined in a warm room standing on an elevated platform. This allows the surgeon to sit comfortably and to take time over the examination. The assessment of uncomplicated primary veins is not usually difficult; as a rule the experienced examiner can deduce where the sites of incompetence are likely to be from the distribution of the varices and a knowledge of the anatomy. Confirmation is by palpation and, if necessary, the tourniquet test [1]. The following plates illustrate some common pattern of varices.

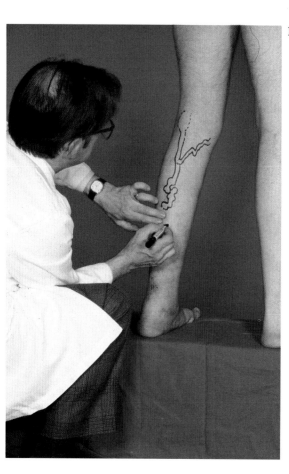

2 This patient has a saphenar varix with incompetence throughout the long saphenous system.

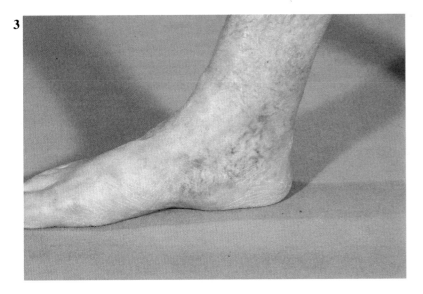

3 A medial ankle flare is diagnostic of an incompetent perforator in the lower calf.

4 Some perforators are clinically obvious.

5 Others are obscured by chronic inflammation and ulceration.

6 Varices on the medial side of the thigh usually stem from saphenofemoral incompetence (see Fig. 26). However, this patient had undergone previous saphenofemoral ligation and this varix was feeding from the femoral vein via perforators at mid-thigh level.

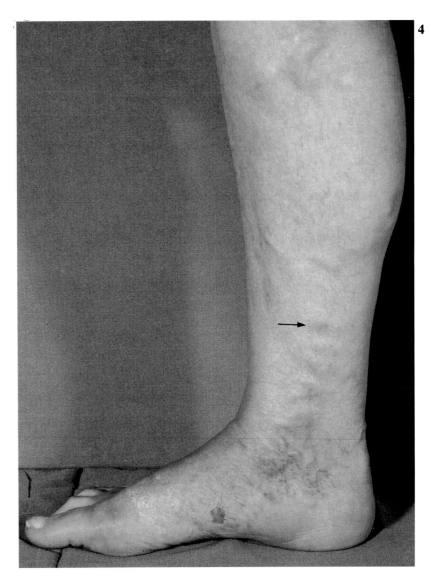

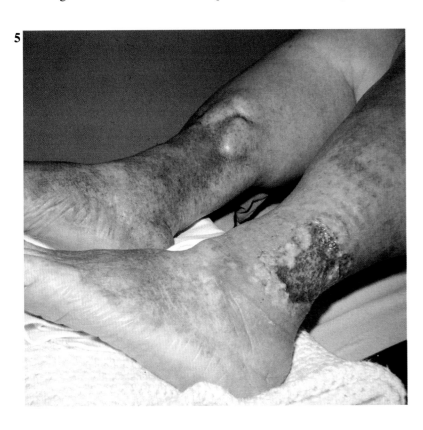

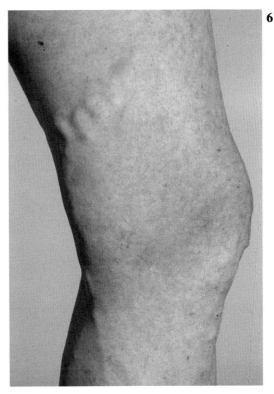

7 Short saphenous incompetence. It is unusual for the incompetent saphenous vein to be so clearly visible.

8 Careful examination is required to determine whether varices behind the knee are fed from the long or short saphenous systems. This patient had an incompetent short saphenous vein which entered the popliteal vein some 10 cm above the joint line.

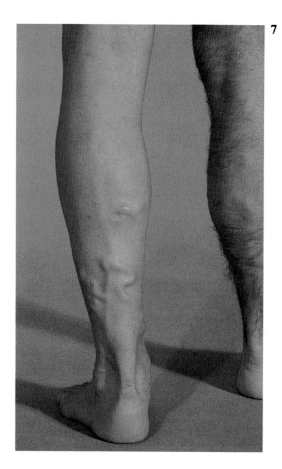

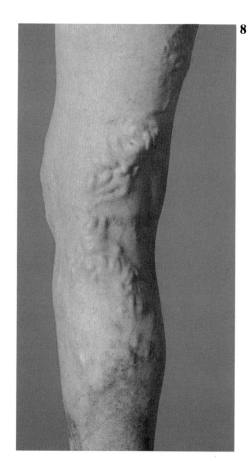

Percussion

9 Percussion is quite helpful in demonstrating connecting channels and confirming incompetence. An impulse felt proximal to the point of percussion simply shows venous continuity. If one percusses proximally and is able to feel an impulse on distal palpation, this indicates valve incompetence in the intervening segment of vein.

Tourniquet test

10 The superficial veins are emptied by elevation and a venous tourniquet is applied to the upper thigh. The patient then stands and the speed and direction of venous filling are observed. Veins filling from below by arterial inflow fill slowly over about half a minute, whereas filling from above by reflux through incompetent deep connections is relatively rapid. By repeating this manoeuvre with the tourniquet moved serially down the leg, the points of incompetence can be mapped out.

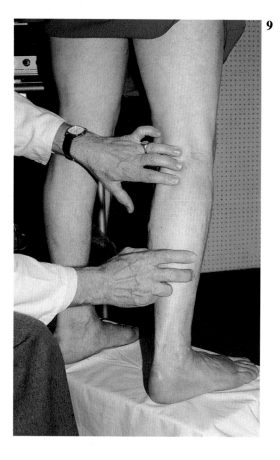

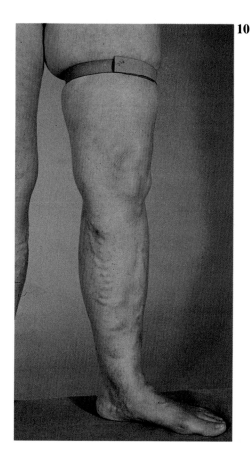

Doppler

There are occasions when simple physical examination is not enough. Even primary varicose veins can be difficult to assess in the obese patient or where there are anatomical variants or developmental abnormalities. The pattern may be obscured by previous operations or sclerotherapy. In the patient with secondary varicose veins inflammation, induration or scarring may make palpation difficult. In such cases Doppler ultrasound examination and phlebography are very helpful.

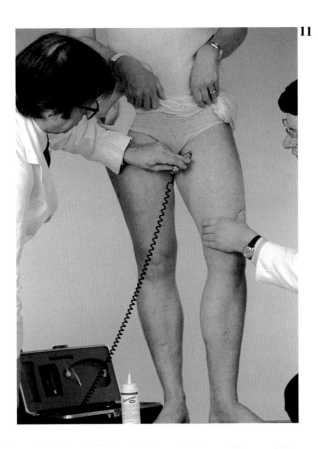

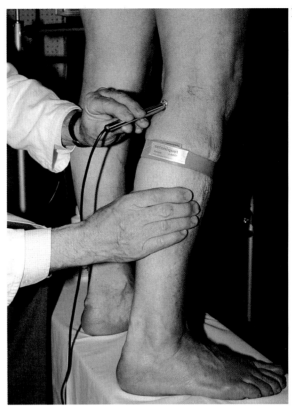

Saphenofemoral reflux

11 The portable Doppler can be used to confirm reflux at sites of incompetence. Here the upper end of the long saphenous vein is insonated while compression is applied at a lower level. A reflux signal is heard on release of the compression. A similar effect can be achieved by asking the patient to perform a Valsalva manoeuvre.

Saphenopopliteal reflux

Saphenopopliteal incompetence is present in one in four patients with varicose veins; the ratio of saphenopopliteal to saphenofemoral incompetence being 1:3 [2].

12 To elicit reflux at the saphenopopliteal junction, the patient is asked to flex the knee slightly. Reflux in the deep system can be distinguished from short saphenous reflux by occluding the latter with a tourniquet or an assistant's finger. In interpreting this test it is important to remember the frequency of variations in the termination of the short saphenous vein [3].

Perforator incompetence

13 Incompetence of perforators can be detected by Doppler, although not with complete accuracy [4]. With the patient either sitting or supine a tourniquet is applied to the calf to prevent reflux down superficial veins; calf compression is applied above the tourniquet while insonating over the area of suspected incompetence.

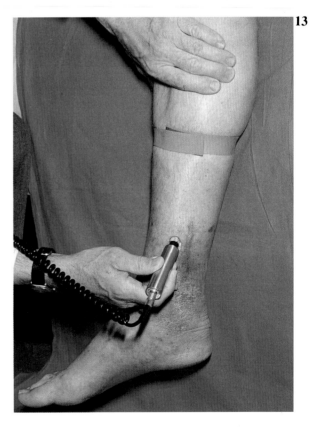

In normal veins blood in the perforators only flows inwards. In varicose veins there is a two-way flux through incompetent perforators during muscular activity. In primary varicose veins the net flow is generally inwards. In chronic venous insufficiency with dysfunction of the deep veins, the net flow is outwards [5].

Deep veins

14 Doppler can also be used as a simple bedside technique to detect deep obstruction or incompetence by insonating over the posterior tibial, popliteal and femoral veins. Spontaneous phasic signals suggest normal flow.

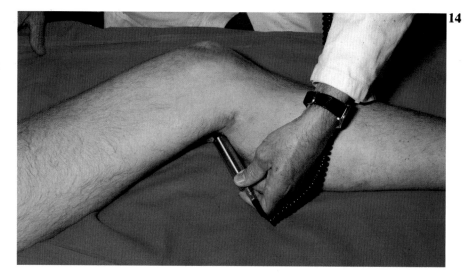

15 Reflux is tested using proximal compression (as shown here) or by Valsalva manoeuvre. Obstruction is tested by applying compression distal to the probe. The technique has been described fully by Barnes [6]. When insonating for reflux, it may be an advantage to have the patient standing.

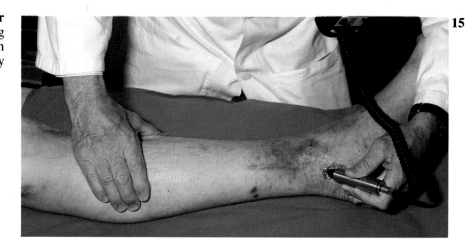

Arterial insufficiency

16 Doppler pedal pressure measurement is valuable where arterial insufficiency is suspected. This patient is being examined in the prone position. The supine position is equally satisfactory (see page 98). The calf attachments were monitoring isotope clearance.

These measurements must be considered in the light of other clinical findings because in the elderly, particularly diabetics with calcified vessels, spuriously high values may be recorded.

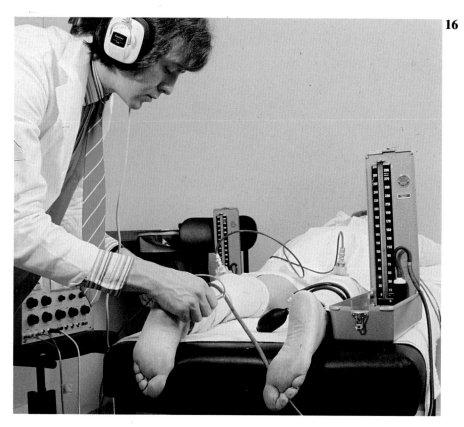

Ambulatory venous pressure

Assessment of the more complex venous problems involves obtaining haemodynamic information about the patency and competence of the deep system and the severity of the venous insufficiency. Excellent surgically relevant descriptions of venous physiology are available [7, 8]. Direct venous pressure measurement is the reference laboratory method. It is still used in research and is the best means of separating the different degrees and patterns of venous insufficiency.

A needle is inserted into a superficial vein on the dorsum of the foot and connected to a manometer. In the normal subject a standard exercise of, for example, twenty steps results in a progressive fall in pressure. Upon resting, the slope of the refilling curve reflects arterial inflow. In the patient with venous outflow obstruction, the pressure may actually rise on exercise. In the patient with incompetent valves in either the deep or the superficial veins, reflux down the leg ensures that the pressure does not fall to the same extent on exercise and the refilling time is short. Whether it is deep or superficial, valve incompetence that is present can be differentiated by repeating the test with a venous tourniquet inflated to 100 mmHg positioned above the knee to exclude long saphenous reflux and just below the knee to exclude short saphenous reflux.

For routine clinical work, however, direct venous pressure measurement has largely been replaced by indirect non-invasive techniques such as foot volumetry [9-11] and the various other types of plethysmography [12-14].

Foot volumetry

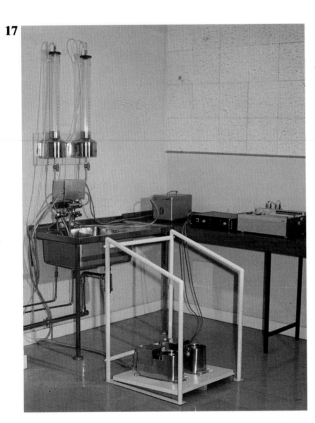

17 The apparatus is essentially a water-filled plethysmograph.

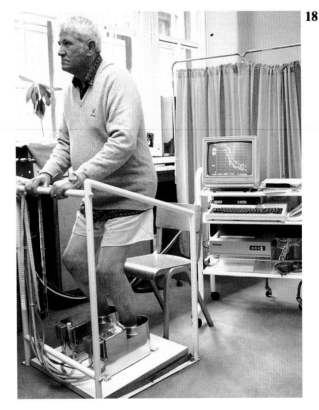

18 The patient stands in two containers that are filled with water at body temperature and maintained at a height of 14 cm from the bottom. The water level is sensed by a photoelectric float sensor, so that changes in foot volume are recorded accurately. The initial foot volume is read from a calibrated reservoir. The patient does a standard series of knee bends to expel blood from the foot and then stands stationary so that venous refilling can be measured. The curve of venous emptying can be seen on the computer screen.

19 The normal foot volumetry tracing is analogous to an ambulatory venous pressure curve. The expelled volume (EV), derived from the distance between baseline and peak, is a measure of the efficiency of the pumps of the calf and foot. The refilling time, expressed as T½ seconds, is a measure of arterial inflow in the normal subject, but in the patient with venous disease it is a measure of valve competence.

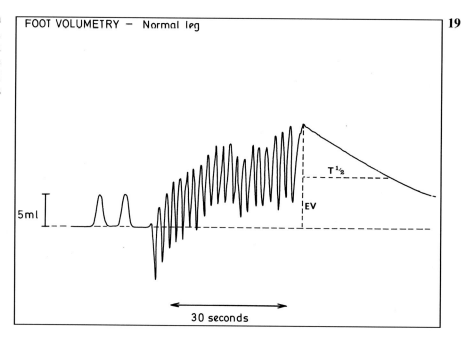

20 A low expelled volume may be the result of obstructed outflow or, as in this case, valve incompetence. The shortened refilling time confirms valve incompetence. As with direct pressure measurement it may be possible to distinguish between deep and superficial incompetence by repeating the test with a thigh and/or calf tourniquet in place to occlude the superficial veins.

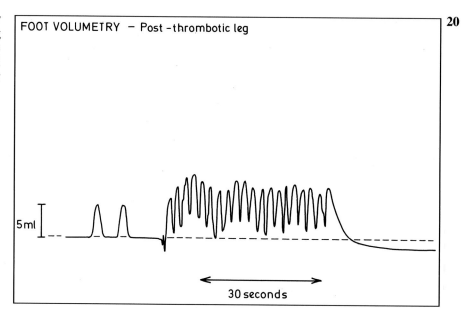

Phlebography

Phlebography remains the most valuable investigation in the management of patients with venous disease. The recent introduction of a new generation of contrast media has been a great step forward[15-17]. These low osmolality agents such as iopamidol (Niopam) and ichexol (Omnipaque) are non-ionic monomeric substances which are less irritating to the vascular endothelium and better tolerated by the patients than previous contrast media. They also produce fewer toxic side effects, thus removing the main objections to this fundamental investigation.

It is essential to select the correct method of phlebography for the particular clinical problem. For a detailed description of

phlebographic techniques the reader is referred to a specialist text[18]. The purpose of this section is to illustrate some typical clinical applications and to point out some common pitfalls.

Uncomplicated primary varicose veins do not require to be investigated by phlebography. In the assessment of chronic venous insufficiency or the post-thrombotic syndrome, unilateral phlebography is usually all that is required. In suspected venous thrombosis both legs should be investigated as a routine, because clinically important thrombus will often be revealed on the asymptomatic side and display of the pelvic veins requires the confluence of boluses of contrast agent from each side.

Ascending phlebography

This is the most generally useful phlebographic technique for detecting acute thrombosis or chronic occlusion of the deep veins. It can also be used to demonstrate incompetent perforators, although varicography has become the preferred method for this indication. It is not the examination of choice for evaluating valve function.

Many different techniques of ascending phlebography have been described. The choice of technique depends on the question the clinician is seeking to answer. The detection of incompetent calf perforators requires careful fluoroscopic monitoring of contrast flow, films being taken at appropriate moments as the veins sequentially are seen to fill. A ruler with radio-opaque markings placed alongside the limb allows a more accurate localisation of the perforators.

When the purpose of the examination is to evaluate venous thombosis, simultaneous bilateral pedal contrast injection is generally the technique chosen, an overcouch radiographic procedure without fluoroscopy. Hand injection is used and tourniquets are placed above the ankle and the knee. The bolus of contrast derived from each leg (50-100 cc per leg) usually allows satisfactory demonstration of the iliac veins and cava. However, ascending phlebography cannot be expected to give adequate visualisation of the pelvic veins and cava in a patient who presents with the signs and symptoms of an occlusive iliofemoral thrombosis.

21 Ascending phlebography displays a large incompetent perforator.

22 In this examination the deep veins have been outlined in the right leg. In the left, because of obstruction to the deep veins, the long saphenous system has filled.

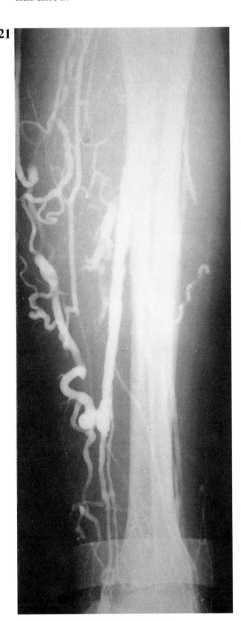

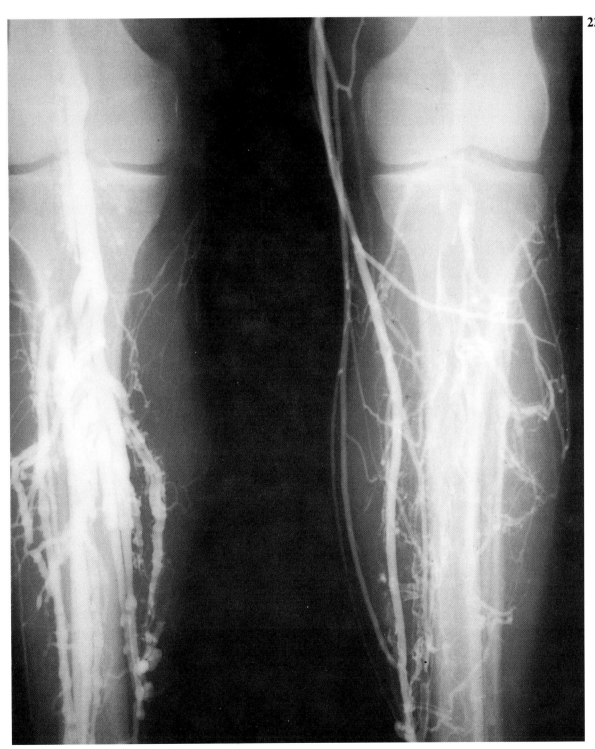

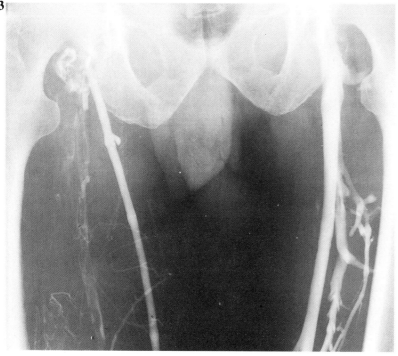

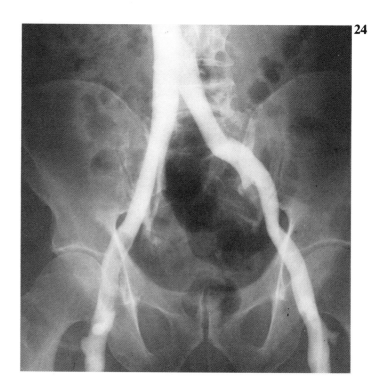

23 In this patient the deep veins of the right leg contain thrombus. The long saphenous vein is therefore acting as collateral while on the left the femoral vein has filled normally.

24 Good visualisation of the iliac veins and cava can be obtained by ascending phlebography, if there is no obstruction to flow. Here, because the thrombus is non-occlusive, it has been possible to define the upper extent of an isolated thrombus of the right external iliac and common femoral veins.

25 The limitations of ascending phlebography in iliofemoral thrombosis are shown here. The lower end of the thrombus in the common femoral vein has been outlined but the more important upper extent cannot be seen.

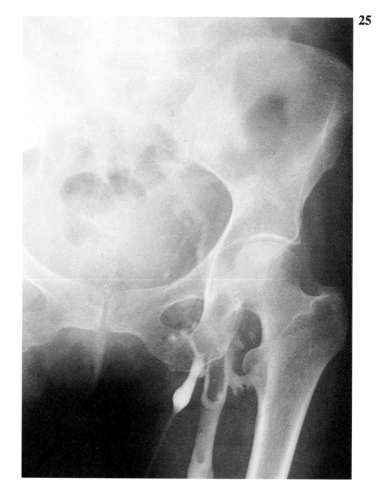

Varicography

This has become the method of choice in the investigation of complicated or difficult veins, notably recurrent varicose veins whose anatomy has been obscured by previous surgery. Contrast medium is injected directly into the varicosities at various levels. A radio-opaque ruler placed alongside the limb aids localisation.

26

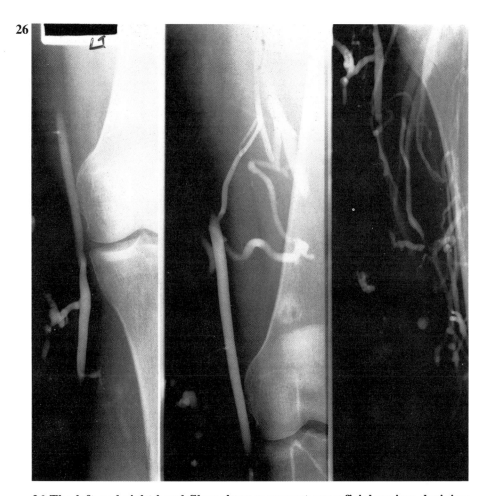

27

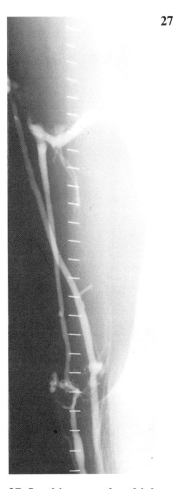

28

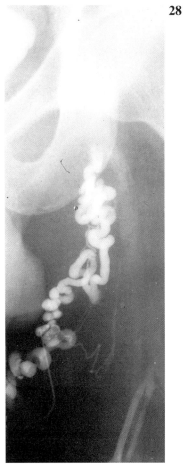

26 The left and right hand films show recurrent superficial varices draining into a remnant of the long saphenous vein. The centre film shows the long saphenous vein terminating at a thigh perforator which drains into a deep femoral vein.

One cannot necessarily be certain from a single film whether this perforator is incompetent. The radiologist may be able to observe reflux on fluoroscopy, otherwise descending phlebography would be necessary to answer the question.

27 In this case the thigh perforator is dilated and clearly incompetent, feeding recurrent varices via the remaining stem of the long saphenous vein.

Note the centimetre marker to assist localisation.

28 This patient has had a previous Trendelenburg operation. Varicography shows that a large varicose vein still connects with the saphenofemoral junction.

Descending phlebography

This is an infrequently used technique which can be helpful in assessing saphenofemoral reflux and deep valve competence. A catheter is positioned in the femoral vein and the patient brought to the erect position. Fluoroscopic monitoring is used to visualise the veins of the upper thigh. Some reflux may occur due to gravity and contrast density but reflux to the knee or below is regarded as abnormal.

29

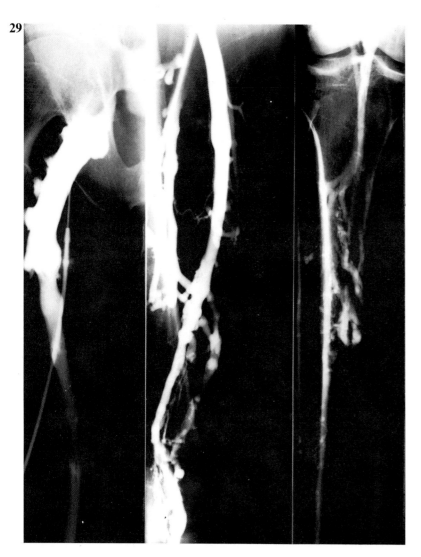

30

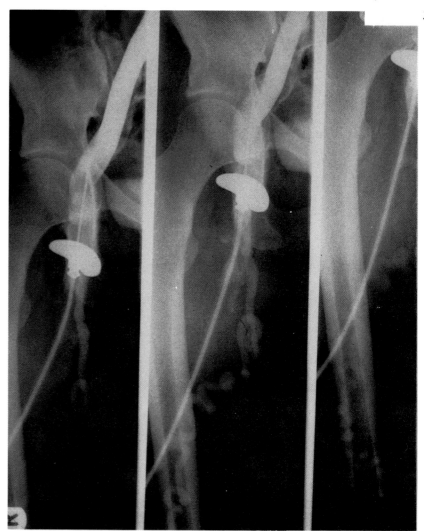

29 The descending method has been used in this patient to detect reflux down the deep system. Contrast material from the perfemoral injection can be seen to have refluxed down the deep and superficial femoral veins and into the calf veins.

30 In this patient with recurrent varices, reflux from the saphenofemoral junction into a thigh varicosity has been demonstrated. Descending phlebography is also the best examination for patients with recurrence appearing to arise in the upper thigh and in whom it is difficult, on physical examination, to decide whether the reflux is occurring at the saphenofemoral junction, thigh perforators or connections with pelvic or epigastric veins.

Pelvic or femoral phlebography

Ascending phlebography may fail to give adequate visualisation of the iliac veins and inferior cava where there is an obstruction to flow, the contrast bolus being delayed and dissipated in collateral veins. In this situation ascending phlebography may be supplemented by pelvic phlebography and, if necessary, a crossover procedure can be performed. In the latter technique a catheter is advanced over the iliac confluence to the opposite side allowing retrograde contrast injection and visualisation of the upper end of the thrombosis.

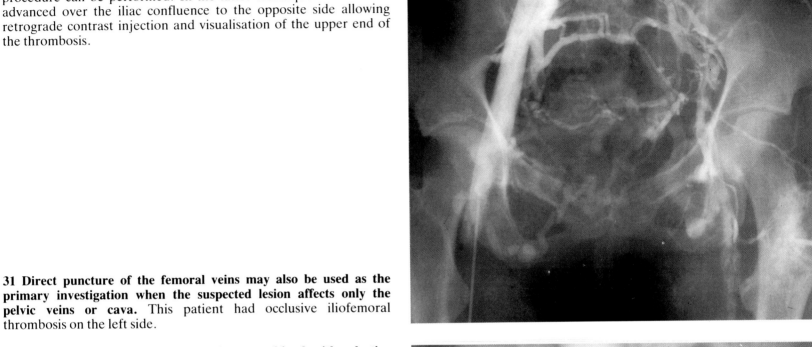

31 Direct puncture of the femoral veins may also be used as the primary investigation when the suspected lesion affects only the pelvic veins or cava. This patient had occlusive iliofemoral thrombosis on the left side.

32 Here the femoral approach has been combined with selective crossover phlebography. An obstructed common femoral vein has prevented the introduction of a cannula from the symptomatic side. It is essential to see the top end of the thrombus to select appropriate treatment.

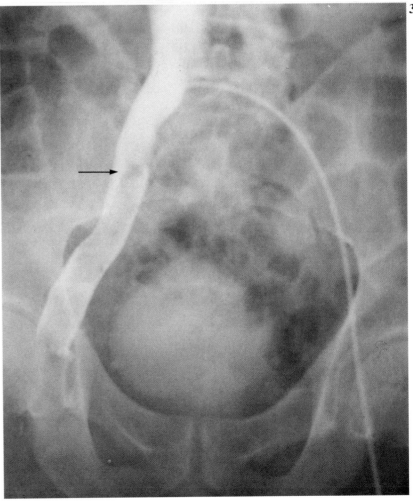

Ultrasound imaging

Modern high resolution ultrasound machines allow direct imaging of the deep and superficial veins of the leg from the upper calf to the inferior vena cava. In addition, pulsed and continuous wave Doppler techniques give information on the presence, direction and quality of blood flow in the veins.

The main applications of the techniques are in the investigation of acute venous thrombosis and chronic venous disease such as valvular incompetence or chronic thrombosis.

In acute venous thrombosis, clot can be seen in the vein lumen although it may be poorly echogenic and therefore difficult to identify; the affected vein shows some compressibility when pressure is applied to it with the ultrasound transducer. This is in contrast to chronic thrombosis where the clot is more echogenic and the vein is completely non-complaint. Collateral vessels may also be identified in chronic thrombosis.

Although flowing blood may be visible on real time ultrasound, much more information on flow can be obtained using Doppler techniques. The direction and velocity of flow can be determined and normal venous flow in the leg veins shows variations with respiration, calf pressure or plantar flexion. The combination of imaging with Doppler velocity measurement means that, theoretically, volume flow can also be calculated in the visualised vessel. In practice the reliability of the values obtained remains in doubt.

In patients with venous occlusion a flow signal may be unobtainable, or, if it is present, the normal variations are lost.

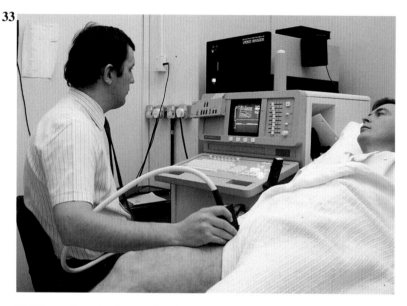

33 The valves in the major leg veins can be visualised directly and their movement during the flow cycle can be assessed. A moderate degree of venous distension is required and this is achieved by performing the examination with the patient lying in the reversed Trendelberg position at 15-30 degrees of tilt. To test valve competence the patient is asked to perform a Valsalva manoeuvre. The femoral vessels are examined first in the supine position and the patient is then turned prone for insonation of the popliteal and distal veins. Some observers prefer to examine the patient standing up.

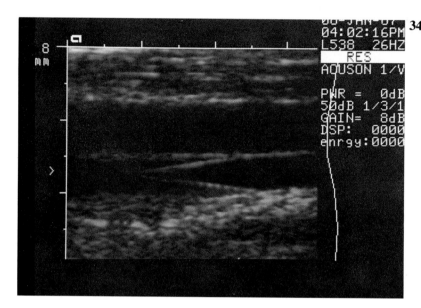

34 This scan shows adjacent superficial femoral artery and vein. The two cusps of a valve are well shown. Doppler techniques are also used for detecting valve incompetence as shown in Figs. **11-15.**

3　Sclerotherapy

Indications

Sclerotherapy became very popular in the 1960s following the work of Fegan[1] and in some centres was used somewhat indiscriminately. It is now clear that it should be used selectively. It is not a direct alternative to surgery. For example, its benefits tend to be shortlived when applied to varices stemming from saphenofemoral or saphenopopliteal incompetence[2-4]. Not only does its use in these circumstances lead to recurrence but it also makes subsequent surgery more difficult. Sclerotherapy has its best place as a treatment of residual or recurrent varices after saphenofemoral and saphenopopliteal incompetence and major perforator incompetence have been dealt with surgically. It may also be suitable as the primary treatment for varices where there is no saphenofemoral or saphenopopliteal reflux, a rare circumstance.

Caution is advised when the indications are purely cosmetic because pigmentation can occur over sclerosed segments.

The lower calf is a particularly hazardous area for sclerotherapy. At this level there is danger of arterial damage and of inducing deep vein thrombosis by the passage of sclerosant through perforators.

Technique

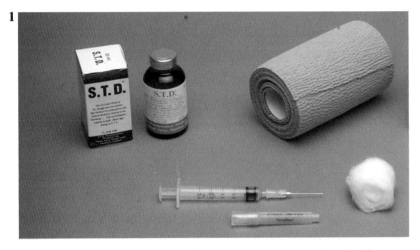

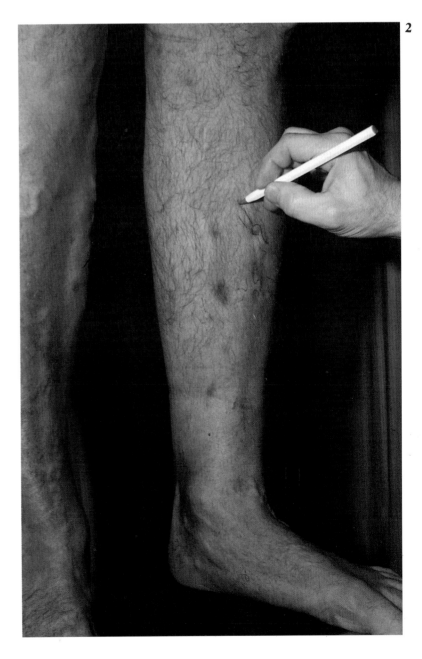

1 For each site to be injected a 2 cc syringe is mounted with 25 gauge needle and loaded with 0.5 cc of sodium tetradecyl sulphate (STD). Compression is applied by means of a high-quality self-adhesive elastic bandage over cotton-wool balls.

2 The veins are marked with the patient standing. The patient then sits with the legs horizontal. The superficial veins will usually fill sufficiently in this position.

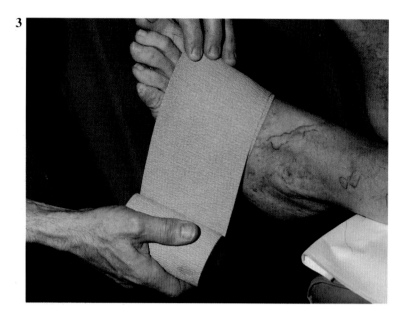

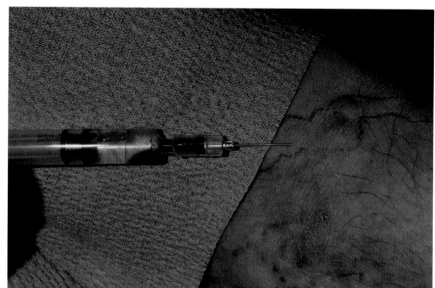

3 The bandage is applied from the base of the toes up to the lowest point of injection.

4 The needle is inserted into the vein and blood drawn back into the syringe. Great care must be taken not to inject into, or adjacent to, an artery. The posterior tibial artery in the lower third of the calf is particularly at risk[5].

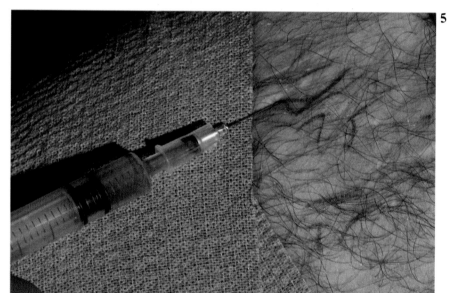

5 The patient lies down and the leg is elevated to empty the veins. During the injection proximal compression is applied with the thumb or fingers to keep the veins empty of blood and temporarily to confine the sclerosant to the injected segment. A cotton-wool ball is applied over the injection point.

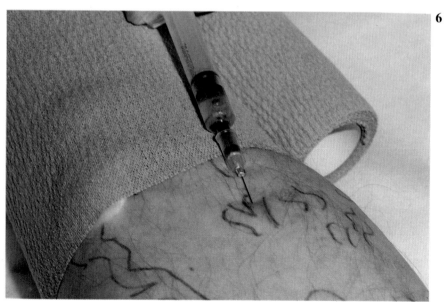

6 The bandage is advanced up to the next point of injection and the procedure repeated. It is the author's practice to limit the number of injections to six.

7 The completed bandage. If a self-adhesive bandage is not available, a graduated elastic stocking should be applied over the bandage to keep the latter in place and sustain the compression.

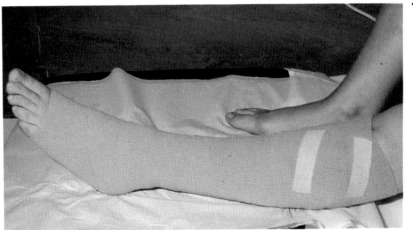

Aftercare

The patient is asked to walk vigorously for 30 minutes immediately and to do an extra 30 minutes walking twice each day. The bandage is left in place undisturbed for 3 weeks. There does not seem to be any advantage in retaining the bandage for longer[6,7]. The patient is asked to report any pain not relieved by simple analgesics. An instruction sheet is provided to reinforce the advice.

On follow up, further injections can be given, if necessary, until a satisfactory effect has been achieved, although it is probably wise to leave an interval of several weeks between treatments.

Complications

8 The direct application of foam sponge (often used as an alternative to cotton wool) to the skin can cause blistering.

Mild to moderate discomfort due to leakage of sclerosant outside the vein is not unusual. Inflammation or ulceration only occur if too much sclerosant has been used and a substantial proportion injected in the superficial tissues. Deep vein thrombosis is also a potential complication. **Strict adherence to the use of small volumes and prompt and regular exercise are important precautions.**

Caution: Severe pain occurring at the time of the injection and propagated down into the foot should raise the possibility of arterial damage. Treatment should be started immediately with heparin and low molecular dextran and the patient admitted to hospital.

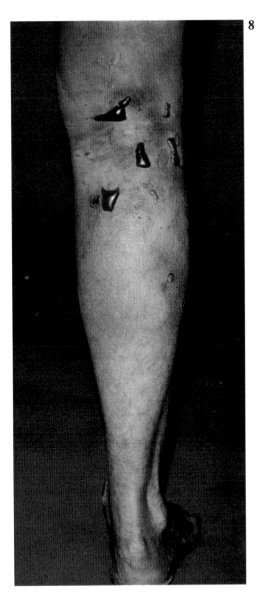

4 Basic Surgical Techniques and the Management of Venous Trauma

Controlling veins

1 When mobilising and controlling veins for repair or anastomosis the use of traumatic instruments, including conventional arterial clamps, should be avoided. Soft-jaw clamps or plastic slings are to be preferred. Fine monofilament arterial sutures are suitable for suturing veins. In the future absorbable sutures may find a useful place in this area of vascular surgery. Standard arterial techniques are appropriate except that when continuous sutures are being used care must be taken not to narrow the lumen by a purse-string effect, the vein wall being thinner and more easily constricted than the arterial wall.

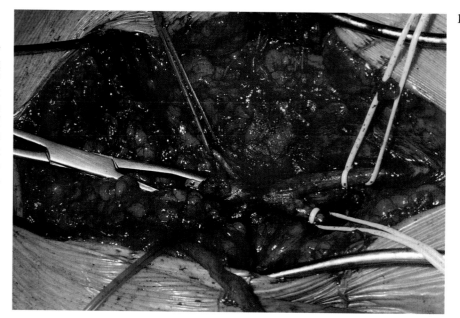

Venous bleeding

2 Haemorrhage from a damaged vein can be more troublesome to deal with than that from an artery, the bleeding point often being difficult to localise. If the haemorrhage is in the region of an important vein, attempts to apply an artery forceps should be avoided unless a discrete bleeding tributary can be seen. The safest method is to control blood loss by pressure around the area and then suture the bleeding point accurately. A lateral tear in a major vein such as an iliac or femoral should be repaired carefully with fine arterial suture, for example 5/0 monofilament, without narrowing the lumen.

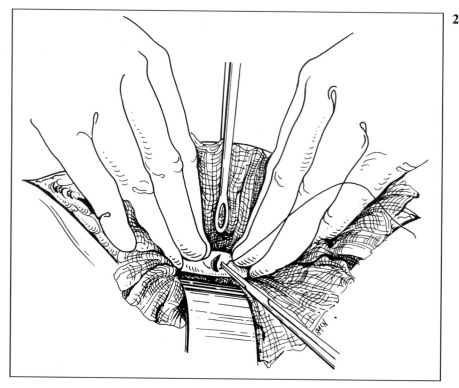

Repair or ligation?

When confronted with more extensive damage to a major vein, the surgeon has a choice between ligation or reconstruction. The issue is controversial. Some authors have argued that, provided it is combined with high elevation of the limb and timely fasciotomy, ligation may be satisfactorily employed without leading to long-term swelling[1,2]. Based on their analysis of the Vietnam Vascular Registry, Rich and colleagues recommended venous reconstruction wherever feasible to reduce early morbidity and long-term swelling[3]. This was supported by other workers particularly in respect of popliteal vein injuries[4,5]. The author's view is that the popliteal vein should be repaired whenever possible. Other veins should be considered on an individual basis taking into account other injuries, the likely availability of collaterals, the degree of contamination of the field and the calibre of surgical expertise available. Veins of the upper limb, the infrarenal cava, external iliac and superficial femoral veins, for example, can usually be ligated with impunity.

3 This patient was trapped between heavy rollers in a paper mill and sustained a shearing and crushing injury to the left shoulder and chest wall. He had a flail segment of chest wall with bilateral pneumothoraces. There was extensive haemorrhage around the shoulder and his left arm was paralysed and ischaemic. The arteriogram showed a severe stenosis of the axillary artery. In addition to his multiple rib fractures, there were fractures to the right clavicle and left scapula.

4 Phlebography showed the axillary vein to be occluded, with visible proximal thrombus. The cephalic vein was noted to bypass the damaged area and was patent. At operation the artery, which was contused and contained an intimal tear, was repaired with a vein patch graft. The brachial plexus was found to be intact. Torn axillary vein could be safely ligated. Postoperatively, the arm was well perfused and there was no swelling or venous congestion.

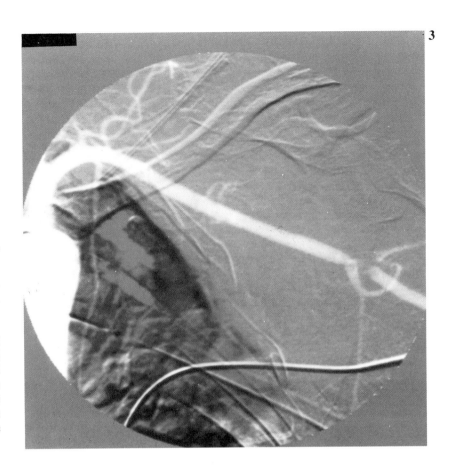

3

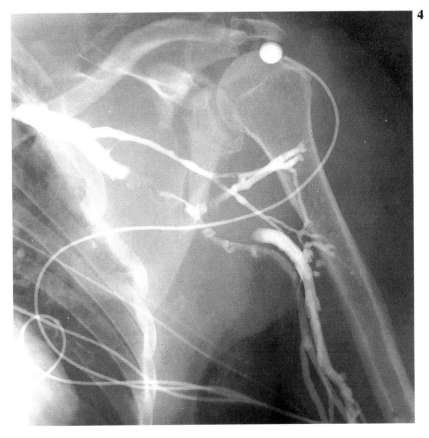

4

Vein replacement

Trauma aside, it is unusual to have to replace a vein. Rare indications would be in association with radical resection of tumour, chronic thrombotic occlusion or the repair of arteriovenous fistula. Venous collaterals are so readily available in most areas of the body that ligation of major veins seldom gives rise to long-term problems of peripheral venous congestion and limb swelling, unless collaterals or lymphatic channels, or both, are also compromised. The use of vein bypass for chronic obstruction is discussed in Chapter 13.

An unresolved issue in venous reconstruction is whether it should be accompanied by arteriovenous fistula. A distal AV fistula may enhance patency by increasing flow. It may, however, add to the morbidity by increasing venous congestion and limb swelling and it also commits the patient to a second operation, 1-2 months later, for closure of the fistula. The author's preference is not to use AV fistula, but to rely on antithrombotic drugs and physical measures to enhance flow.

If replacement is required, what material should be used? The saphenous vein is the graft of choice. The cephalic vein is a possible substitute, although it is likely to have to be modified as a panel graft to obtain sufficient calibre. If a vein of larger calibre is required, the internal jugular can be substituted although being very thin-walled, it is much less easy to handle than the limb veins.

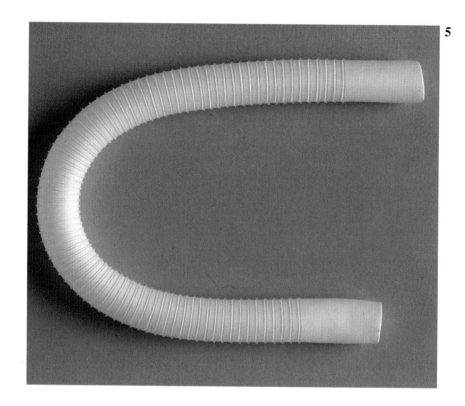

5 Synthetic replacement of vein is only required in exceptional circumstances. Externally supported PTFE (polytetrafluoroethylene) is currently the materal of choice[6]. Thin-walled PTFE can also be used to patch major veins[7].

Panel graft

If it is necessary to replace a vessel of the diameter of a femoral, iliac or portal vein a suitable graft can be constructed by joining two or more lengths of saphenous or cephalic vein longitudinally. This is known as a 'panel graft' and is described step by step below.

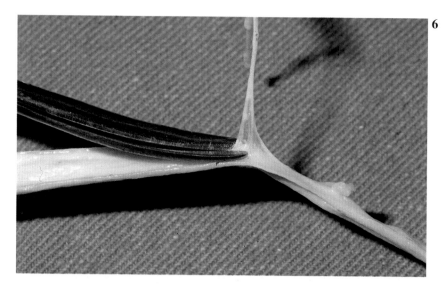

6 A portion of long saphenous vein has been removed and is being cleaned of loose adventitia.

7 The two segments to be joined are slit longitudinally.

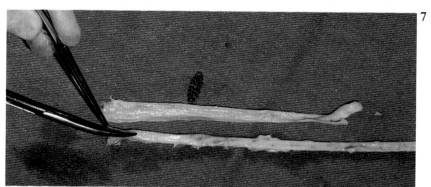

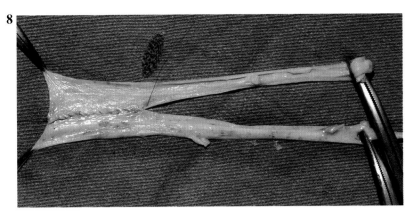

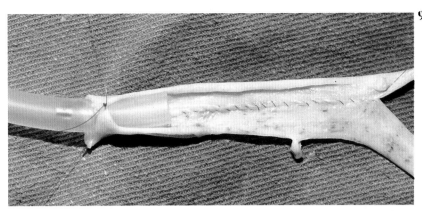

8 They are joined with a running monofilament.

9 The graft is formed into a tube over a stent.

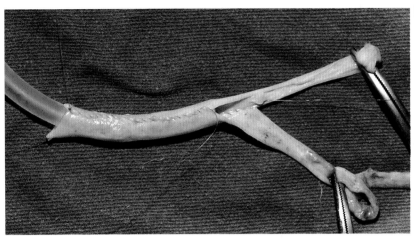

10 Here the anterior wall of the graft is being completed over the stent.

11 An alternative technique is to wrap a vein spirally around a stent. It is then converted into a tube with a running monofilament.

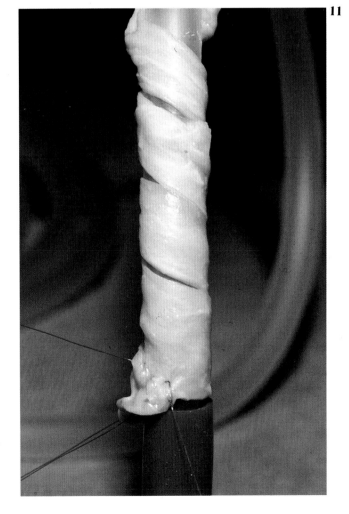

Postoperative care

When a venous reconstruction or repair has been carried out, there is a tendency to postoperative thrombosis. The risk can be minimised by a week's course of intravenous heparin or 500 cc of low molecular weight dextran daily for three days. A three month's course of warfarin is also recommended. **With both heparin and oral anticoagulants careful control should be exercised and anticoagulation maintained on the low side of the therapeutic range, because haematoma can nullify the benefits of surgery.**

Physical measures are very important. High elevation of the affected limb is maintained in the early postoperative period. Active ankle and foot exercises are encouraged. Intermittent pneumatic compression can be applied to enhance flow in the deep veins and graduated elastic compression hosiery is fitted before mobilisation. It is continued for as long as there is any tendency to leg swelling.

5   Primary Varicose Veins(Part 1)

The organisation of care

The patient with uncomplicated varicose veins, provided that he or she is in good health, is ideally suited for day care. The many advantages of this type of care have been well documented[1-7]. In this context the careful assessment of the patient in the outpatient clinic is vital; both in terms of the venous disease and of the patient's general health and social circumstances[8].

Saphenofemoral ligation

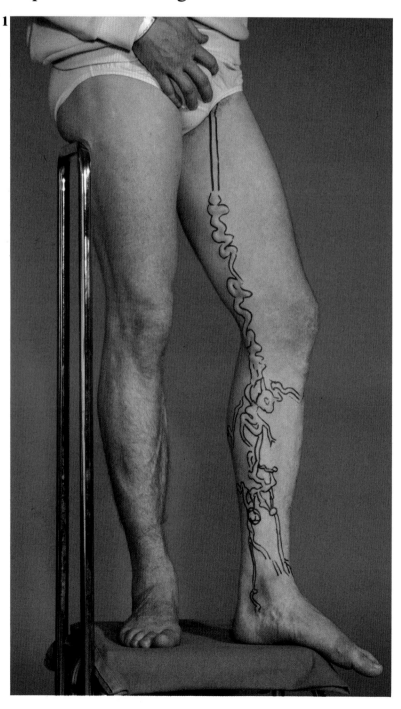

Surgery for primary varicose veins

Most operations have four principal aims:
1 Control of proximal incompetence at the saphenofemoral and/or the saphenopopliteal junction.
2 Removal of the stem by which reflux is transmitted to tributaries.
3 Interruption of incompetent perforators.
4 Removal of the principal varicosities.

1 As in all varicose vein operations the legs are marked beforehand by the surgeon who is to carry out the operation.

2 This operation is otherwise known as the Trendelenburg procedure, high ligation, or juxtafemoral ligation. Like other operations on the veins of the lower limbs (with the exception of thrombectomy), it is carried out with the table tilted head down.

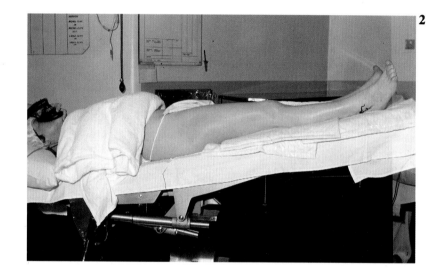

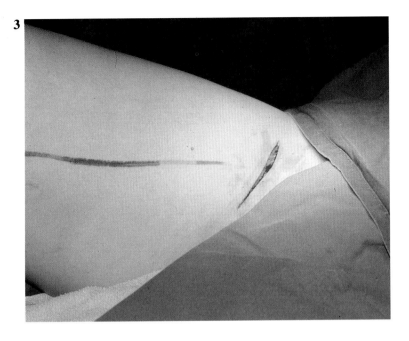

3 A 6-8 cm incision is centred on a point 3-4 cm below and lateral to the pubic tubercle where the long saphenous vein pierces the cribiform fascia to join the femoral vein.

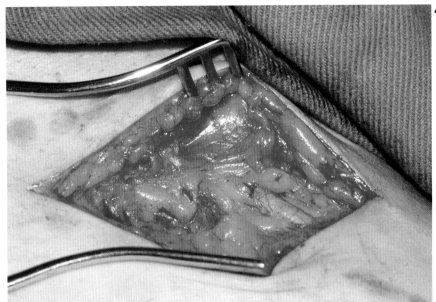

4 The incision is deepened through the membranous layer of the superficial fascia. The upper end of the long saphenous vein comes into view in the medial part of the wound.

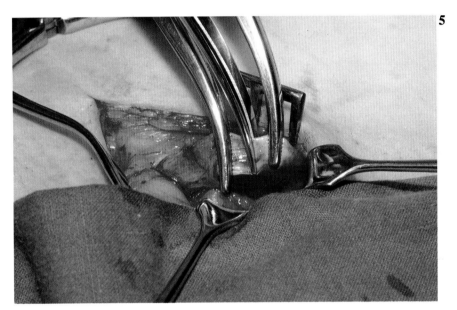

5 In thin individuals the femoral vein and artery may lie close to the surface. It is not unknown for one of them to be divided in mistake for the saphenous vein. PROVIDED THAT THERE IS NO DOUBT OF ITS IDENTITY, the saphenous vein is picked up between Mayo's forceps and divided. This greatly facilitates dissection of the tributaries and display of the saphenofemoral junction.

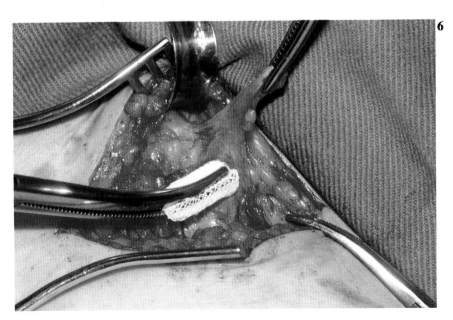

6 Here the saphenous vein, having been divided, has been turned upwards. A dissecting pledget is being used to define the anatomy.

Normally there should be at least three tributaries: the superficial external pudendal, the superficial inferior epigastric and the superficial circumflex iliac veins (see Chapter 1, Fig. **6**). **It is not enough to ligate these tributaries at the point where they join the long saphenous vein. They should be dissected well clear of the junction, at least to the first bifurcation, to ensure that no connections are present which could give rise to recurrence.**

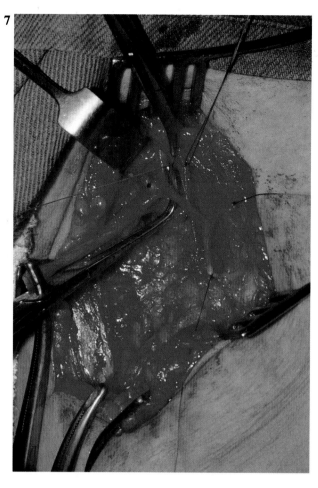

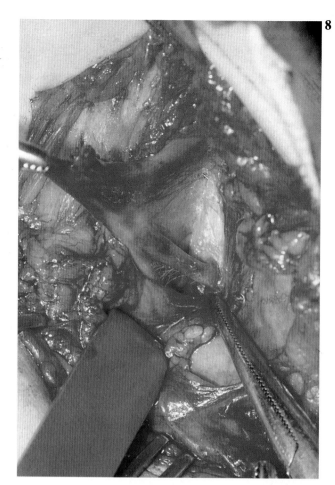

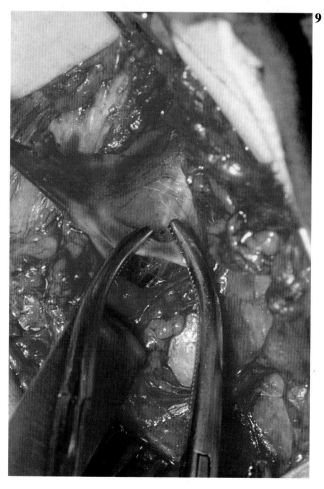

7 In this operation on the left saphenofemoral junction (a different operation from that shown in the previous illustration), the divided stump of the long saphenous vein is being held downwards and medially. A ligature is being passed around the proximal part of the superficial circumflex iliac vein. The superficial external pudendal and the superficial inferior epigastric veins have yet to be dissected out but on the right of the picture the superficial circumflex iliac vein has been dissected well beyond its bifurcation and its two tributaries ligated separately with synthetic absorbable ligatures.

This is an example of the anatomical abnormality shown in Chapter 1, Fig. **8**, whereby the anterolateral thigh vein joined the superficial circumflex iliac, so that a single ligation close to the saphenofemoral junction would have left the iliac and thigh branches in continuity and thus predisposed to recurrence.

8 The saphenous vein stump is being held up in forceps. The superficial external pudendal artery has been ligated and divided where it crossed the femoral vein immediately below the junction. This allowed incision of the fascia of the lower edge of the foramen ovale and exposure of the femoral vein for a distance of 2-3 cm above and below the junction, so that all tributaries which might give rise to recurrence could be ligated. This should include the deep external pudendal vein (indicated by lower forceps) which joins the femoral vein or the long saphenous vein at the medial side of the junction.

9 Ligation of the deep external pudendal vein. Haemostats have been placed on the vein before division. This step must be carried out with care as avulsion gives rise to bleeding which may be difficult to control (see Chapter 4, Fig.**2**).

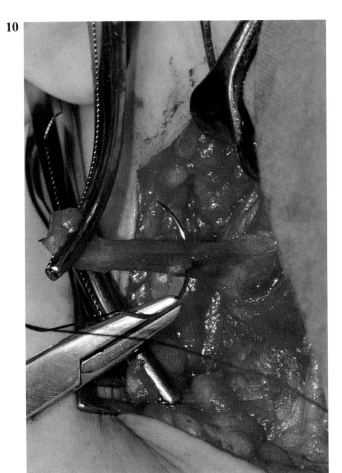

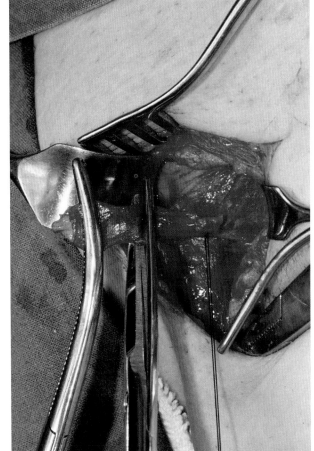

10 All tributaries having been ligated, the long saphenous vein is transfixed approximately 1 cm clear of the femoral. The position of the ligature is important because it must not cause narrowing of the femoral vein nor yet give rise to a *cul de sac* in which thrombus might form.

11 The ligated vein is trimmed back leaving a generous stump to ensure that the ligature cannot slip.

12 An important manoeuvre after saphenofemoral ligation is to search for upper thigh tributaries, notably the posteromedial superficial femoral vein. The knee is well flexed and, with finger dissection, the distal end of the divided long saphenous vein followed as far as possible down the thigh.

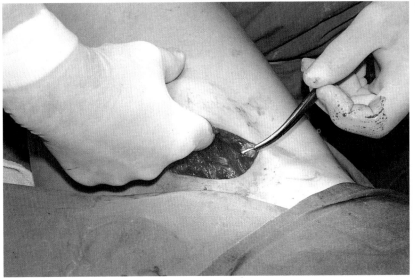

13 Usually, by retraction on the lower edge of the wound, the posteromedial vein can be clipped and ligated.

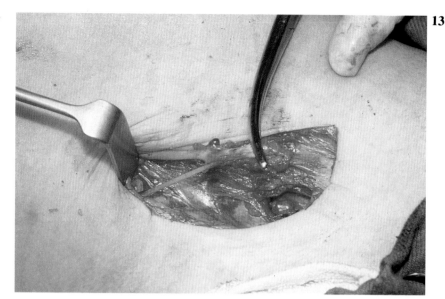

14 Alternatively, a very small incision can be made over the finger tip, the saphenous vein drawn out and the posteromedial vein ligated at this point. This not only reduces the likelihood of recurrence, but also minimises haematoma in the upper thigh after stripping.

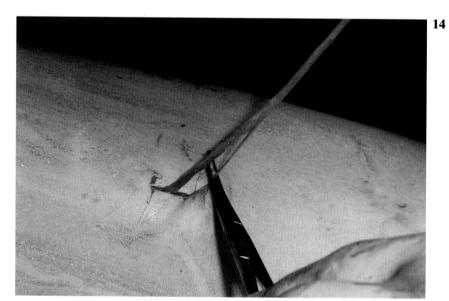

15 The wound is closed with subcutaneous and subcuticular 3/0 synthetic absorbable suture. This operation may be combined with stripping, in which case the end of the skin stitch is left unknotted to allow removal of the stripper.

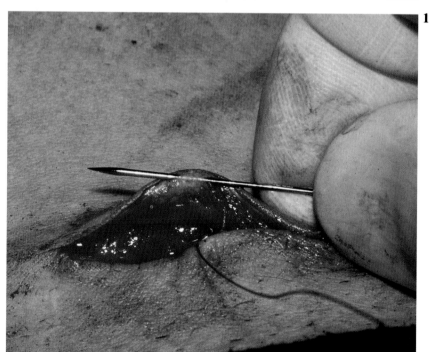

Pitfalls of saphenofemoral ligation

There are a number of pitfalls in varicose vein surgery, some of which arise from the anatomical variations which are frequently found in this region, hence the need for careful dissection to expose completely the saphenofemoral junction and the adjacent femoral vein.

16 A relatively common example. At first sight it looked like a straightforward dissection. What appeared to be the saphenous vein was picked up with forceps and divided.

17 Further dissection showed that there were two saphenous veins, the medial one being more correctly identified as a large high posteromedial vein.

18 Both trunks required to be ligated. After this the saphenofemoral junction was dissected out in the manner described earlier.

Damage to the femoral vein or femoral artery are well recognised complications[9,10]. They may occur because of failure to recognise anatomical structures or because of inept attempts to deal with haemorrhage. **Serious haemorrhage should be controlled in the first instance by tilting the table head further down and by applying local pressure.** The bleeding point is eventually repaired accurately under direct vision (see Chapter 4, Fig. 2).

Caution: If there is technical difficulty or suspicion of damage to a main femoral vessel, the help of a vascular surgeon should be sought immediately.

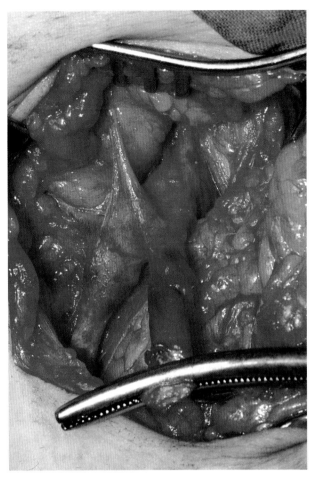

16

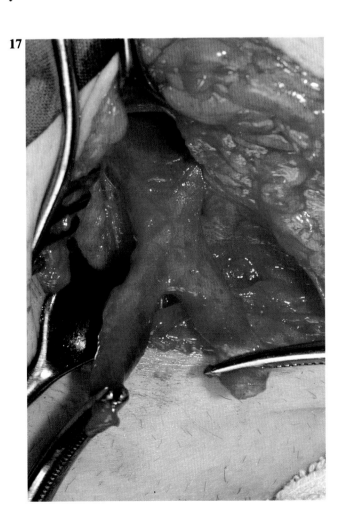

17

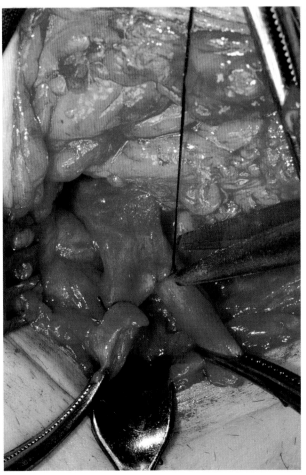

18

Saphenopopliteal ligation

The importance of accurate pre-operative assessment cannot be overemphasised because it determines the position of the patient on the operating table and also the level of the incision. Patients with short saphenous incompetence may also have incompetence of the long saphenous system (page 21). If the patient is relatively thin and supple, satisfactory access to the popliteal fossa can be achieved in the supine position, but in most cases it is necessary to turn the patient face down after the long saphenous has been dealt with. The knee is slightly flexed, to relax the hamstrings and the popliteal fascia, by placing a sandbag under the ankle.

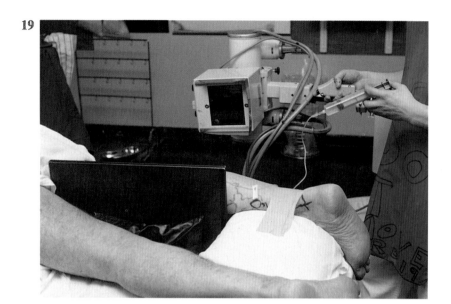

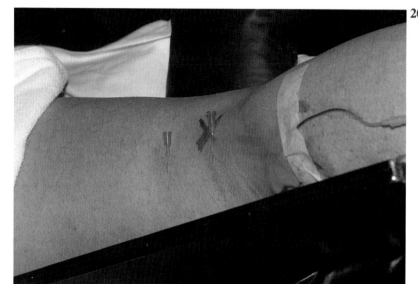

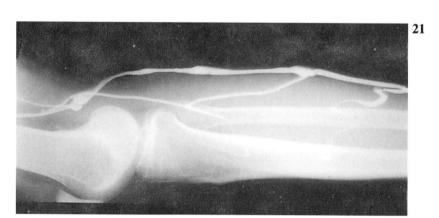

19 A number of authors have emphasised the variations in termination of the short saphenous vein[11-14]. Because a transverse incision is advisable behind the knee, which limits access, Hobbs has advocated phlebography which can be done pre-operatively, in the anaesthetic room or at any stage during the operation[15].

20 A cannula is placed in the short saphenous vein in the lower calf and 10-20 ml of non-ionic contrast medium injected. If the patient is conscious a Valsalva manoeuvre should be performed; if the patient is asleep, the respiration should be momentarily halted at the time of the injection to obtain satisfactory filling of the popliteal vein, both proximal and distal to the junction. The two fine blue needles are placed as radiological markers.

21 A single lateral view is all that is required.

22 A transverse incision of 6-8 cm is centred over the saphenopopliteal junction. If phlebography has not been done and there is uncertainty as to the precise site of the junction, the incision should be placed about a finger's breadth proximal to the skin crease.

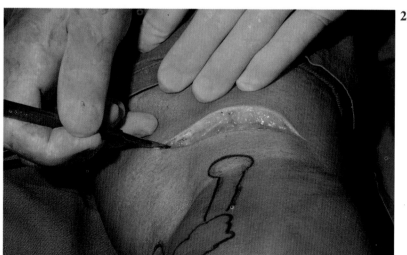

23 The short saphenous vein at this level is under the deep fascia, which is incised longitudinally.

24 The vein is not always easy to find and the area must be searched thoroughly, particularly towards the lateral side.

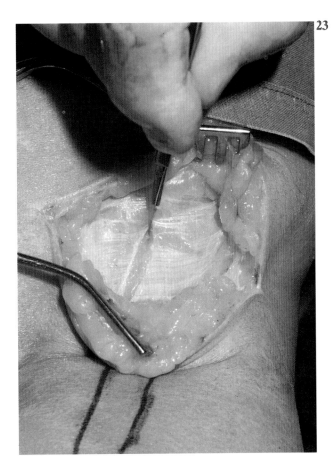

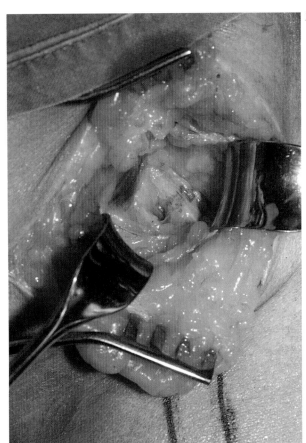

25 Assisted by knee flexion to relax the structures in the fossa the short saphenous vein is mobilised for division between haemostats. This dissection is best done with a mounted pledget. Note the popliteal vein beneath.

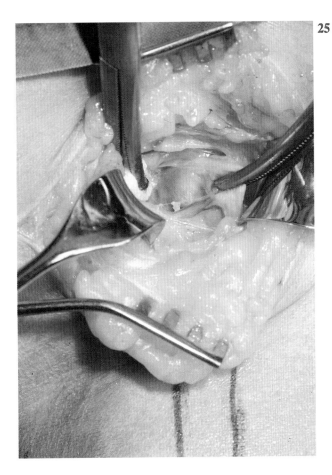

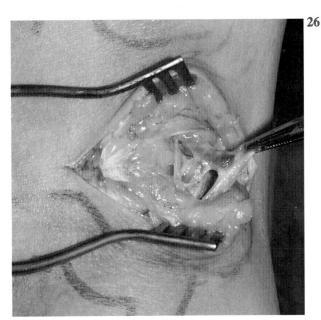

26 Here, in a different patient, the short saphenous vein is lifted up to facilitate dissection of the junction. The medial and lateral popliteal nerves or their branches may have to be mobilised carefully to give across to the junction.

Caution: These nerves are at risk if adequate exposure is not obtained.

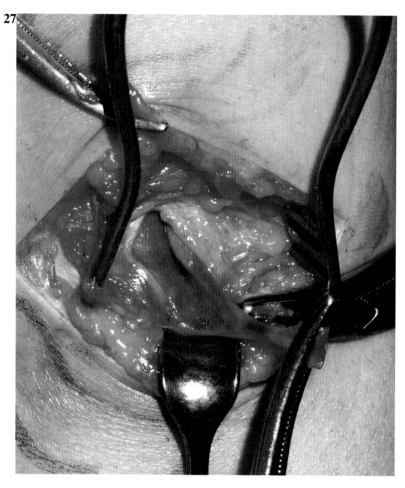

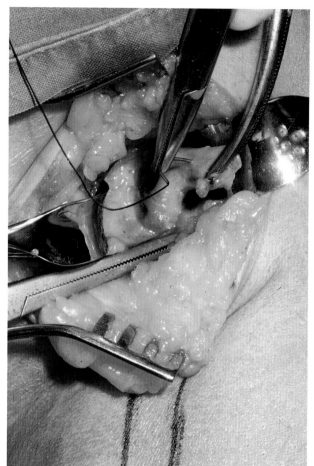

27 The dissection has been carried deeper. The medial popliteal nerve can be seen to the left of the popliteal vein. The stump of the short saphenous vein is drawn down and to the right, displaying tributaries requiring ligation. Their number is quite variable. Particularly important are the posterior thigh vein (Chapter 1, Fig. **10**), which here is held in the upper haemostat behind the arm of the retractor, and the connection with the posteromedial tributary of the long saphenous vein.

28 The short saphenous vein is transfixed and flush ligated with synthetic absorbable suture. Where the short saphenous vein is seen to enter a gastrocnemial vein, the latter is best left intact (unless the patient has a gastrocnemius syndrome—see page 18) and the short saphenous ligated distal to the point of entry.

It is not the author's practice to strip the short saphenous vein.

29 The deep fascia is closed with 3/0 synthetic absorbable suture.

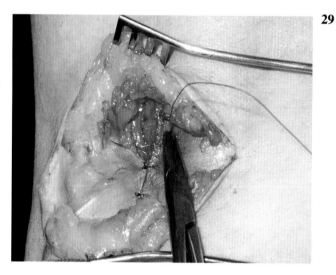

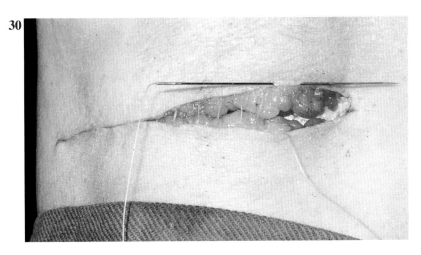

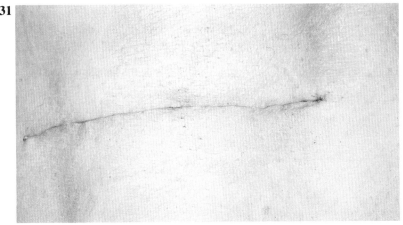

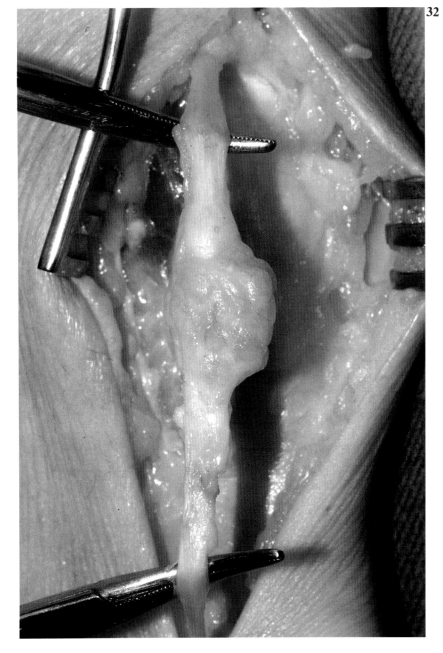

30 The skin is closed with subcuticular suture of the same material.

31 The completed closure.

32 The sural nerve can be readily damaged during varicose vein surgery. This figure shows a dissection of a sural nerve neuroma in a patient who complained of a hypersensitive scar with pain and parasthesiae radiating to the lateral border of the foot.

6 Primary Varicose Veins (Part 2)

Stripping

Fashions have changed considerably over recent years concerning the need for and the technique of stripping. Study of patients with recurrent varicose veins suggests that stripping of the long saphenous vein at the original operation would, in many cases, have reduced the likelihood and the extent of recurrence by removing the stem through which residual points of incompetence in the groin or thigh connect with distal veins (see page 27). This view is supported by a controlled trial[1].

Because perforators in the calf, unlike those in the thigh, seldom connect directly with the long saphenous vein and because the reported incidence of saphenar nerve damage ranges between 23 and 58 per cent[1,2], there is no clear case for stripping in the calf below the junction of the posterior arch vein with the long saphenous. If the stripping is confined to the thigh portion, the incidence of saphenous neurological symptoms is reported to be less than 5 per cent[3]. Different opinions also exist as to whether the vein should be stripped upwards or downwards. Proponents of downward stripping believe that haemostasis is better if the tributaries are pulled downwards before being disrupted and that nerve damage is less[2,4]. The alternative view is that nerve damage is unlikely if stripping is confined to the thigh and that upward stripping allows the stripper to be followed up with firm bandaging to minimise haematoma. The author's preference is to strip upwards from a point between 5 cm and 10 cm below the knee joint.

Technique

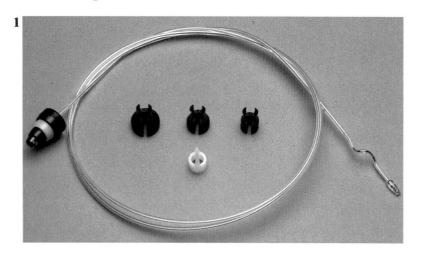

1 A disposable stripper is preferred which allows the 'acorn' to be attached to either end.

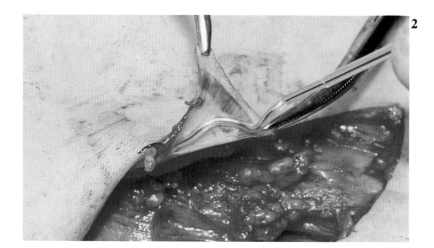

2 The saphenofemoral ligation having been completed, the stripper is passed down to the region of the junction of the posterior arch vein with the long saphenous between 5 cm and 10 cm below the line of the knee joint. Using the stripper as a guide, the long saphenous is exposed through a small skin-crease incision.

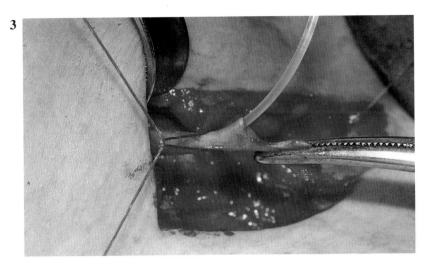

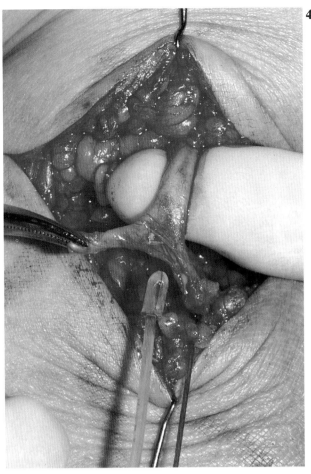

3 The vein is tied on to the stripper in the groin.

4 If there is any difficulty in threading the stripper down, it can be passed up from below. Here the long saphenous vein has been exposed just below the knee.

5 The stripper is easier to insert if an opening is made in the side of the vein rather than transecting it.

6 The distal long saphenous and the arch veins having been ligated, the stump of the saphenous to be removed has been tied on to the stripper. An acorn appropriate to the size of the vein is attached and pulled below the skin, which is closed with an absorbable subcuticular or a monofilament skin suture.

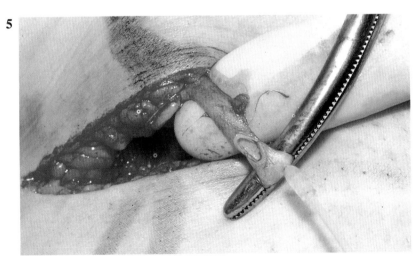

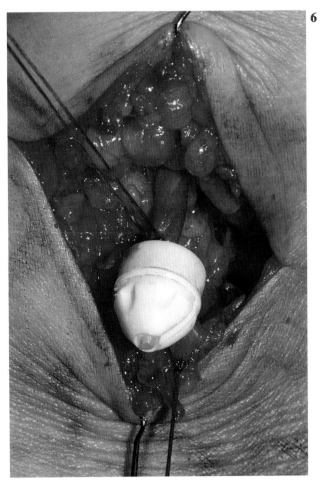

7 The groin wound is then closed, except for the last knot, leaving the stripper protruding. The remainder of the operation (that is avulsions or ligations at other sites in the leg) is completed. The leg is elevated. The bandage follows the stripper up the leg as the vein is stripped out through the groin wound whose final knot is then tied.

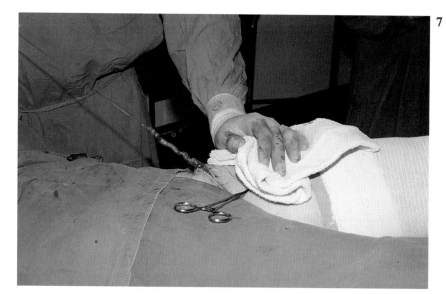

Removal of the long saphenous vein without a stripper

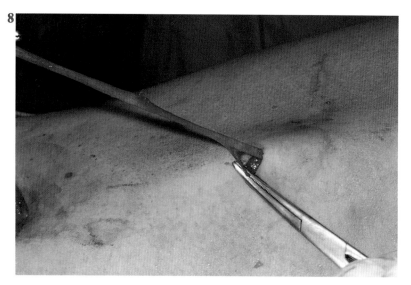

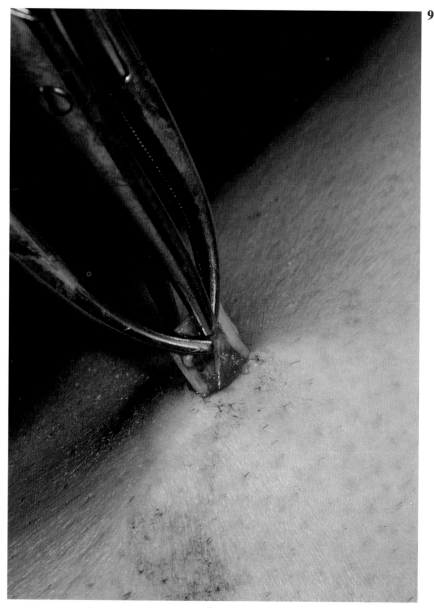

8 It is not essential to use a stripper to remove the long saphenous vein. If there are incompetent perforators or major tributaries in the thigh, it is the author's preference to remove the long saphenous vein through a few 1-2 cm incisions.

9 These incisions are placed over junctions or blow-outs to allow ligation of the connecting veins. This technique is particularly preferred if it is intended to continue the operation in the lower leg under tourniquet (see page 54).

Removal of varices

Avulsion method

Varices may be eradicated by dissection-ligation or by avulsion. The latter technique has steadily gained in popularity in recent years and has cosmetic advantages because it can be carried out through very small incisions. The author's preference in the case of primary varicose veins is to deal with the majority of the varices by the avulsion technique of 'multiple cosmetic phlebectomy'[5].

In some patients with primary varicose veins there is no need specifically to interrupt perforators (see Chapter 2, Fig. **13**). However, where large perforators have been detected and particularly if there are signs of venous insufficiency affecting the skin or subcutaneous tissues, perforators should be ligated on or under the deep fascia.

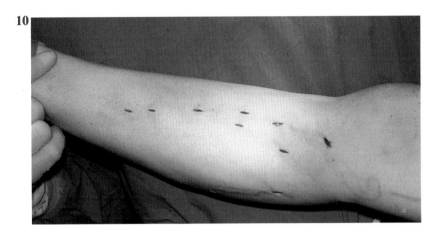

10 The proximal sources of reflux having been dealt with, a tourniquet is applied (see Chapter 7). The remaining varices are removed through a series of miniature incisions of approximately 1 cm in length.

11 If a tourniquet is not used, bleeding is controlled by elevation of the leg and local pressure.

12 Another effective way of reducing haemorrhage is to suspend the leg from a dripstand. The whole operation can be performed with the leg in this position, although it is less convenient for access.

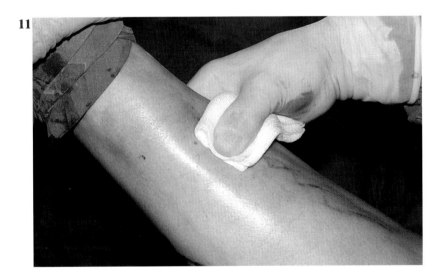

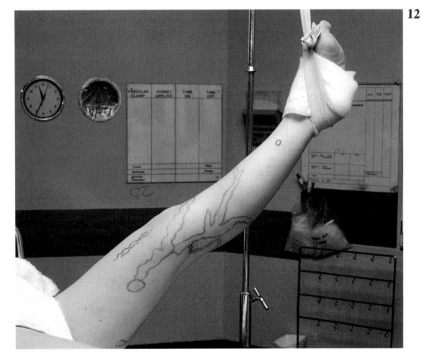

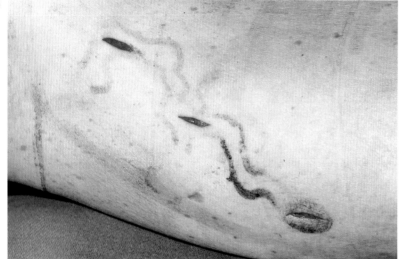

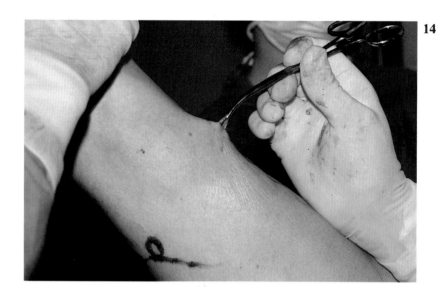

13 Veins are marked with circles or 'tramlines' so that the incision can be made in unmarked skin to avoid tattooing the scar with pigment. The incisions are placed longitudinally and sufficiently close together so that the entire intervening section(s) of each vein can be removed.

14 The vein is grasped with a mosquito forceps and gently 'winkled' out.

15 Surprisingly long lengths of vein can be removed by this method.

16 Complete segments of vein are removed between adjacent incisions.

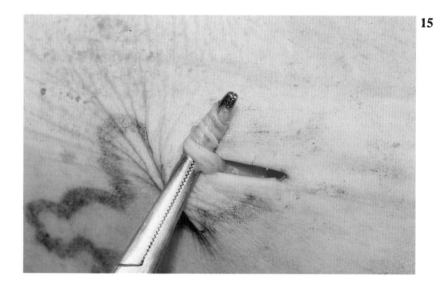

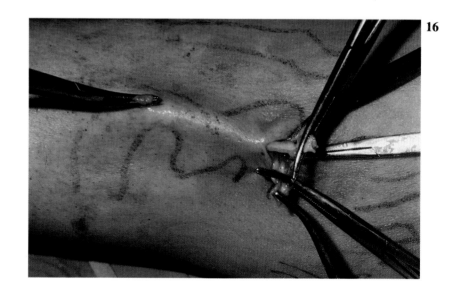

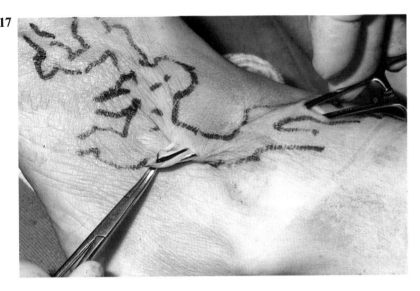

17 Here varices on the foot are being removed.

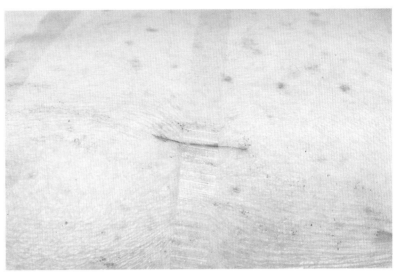

18 These wounds can be closed with single skin sutures, absorbable subcuticular sutures or with adhesive strips, achieving very satisfactory cosmetic results.

Dissection ligation

19 This method is preferred for dealing with large incompetent perforators. The perforator having been carefully marked pre-operatively, an incision sufficient to admit the tip of the little finger is made over the mark. Dissection is carried down to the deep fascia where the perforator can be felt passing through a fascial opening. By sweeping around with the finger at the level of the deep fascia, other perforators can be sought over a wide area.

20 The perforator is ligated or, if it is some distance from the incision, clipped. The wound is closed as described above.

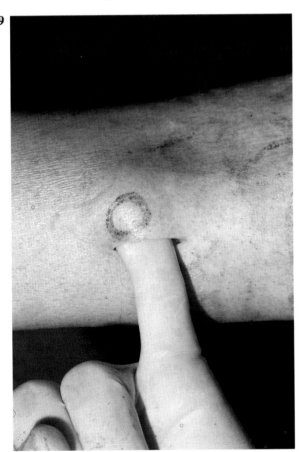

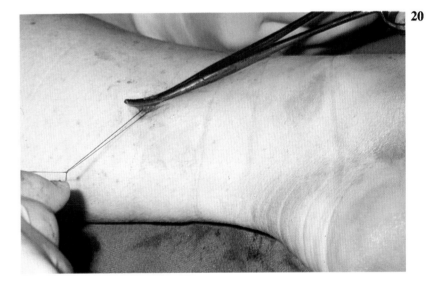

7 The Use of Tourniquets

A tourniquet can be a most useful adjunct to varicose vein surgery, especially in recurrent varicose veins or where previous sclerotherapy or inflammation makes dissection difficult.

1 If saphenofemoral ligation is required this is done first, together with any further dissection that may be needed in the thigh. The leg is then exsanguinated with a sterile Esmarch bandage. If stripping is intended, the Esmarch can be applied while the stripper is *in situ* so that removal of the saphenous vein can be left as the final manoeuvre of the operation, after the leg has been bandaged. Alternatively, the author's preference is to strip out the long saphenous vein before application of a tourniquet. The vein is taken out through a series of miniature thigh incisions, down to the level of the tibial condyles, with individual ligature of the tributaries thus minimising haematoma formation. This method is described in Chapter 6.

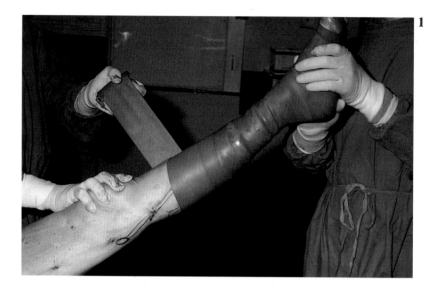

2 A second Esmarch is applied around the mid thigh. After removal of the first Esmarch bandage, the subsequent dissection is performed in a bloodless field. In the case of avulsions no elevation or manual compression is necessary. The leg is bandaged before the tourniquet is released

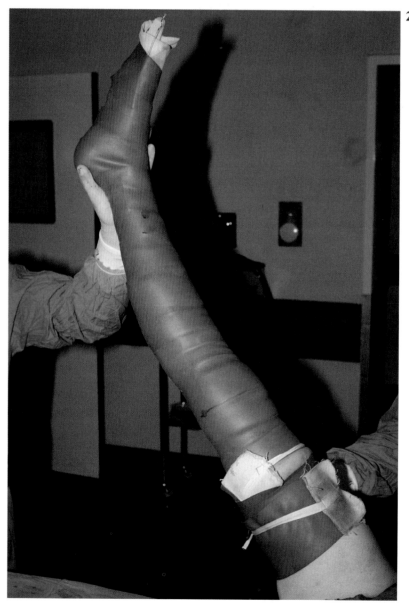

3 A better method of applying a tourniquet to the limb is to combine the Rhys-Davies exsanguinator with a pneumatic tourniquet. The surgeon can then be certain that the tourniquet is exerting the correct pressure for safe control. However, if initial surgery in the groin or thigh is required, it becomes necessary to re-prepare the skin and re-drape because the pneumatic tourniquet cannot be sterilised conveniently.

The Rhys-Davies exsanguinator consists of a sausage-like double-layered inflated rubber tube. The assistant rolls it up his arm and grasps the patient's foot.

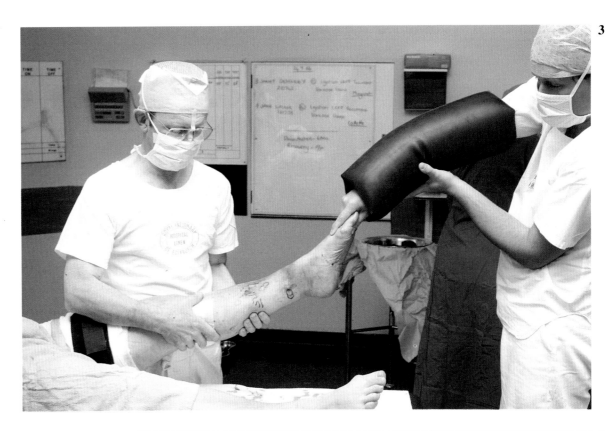

4 The assistant rolls the exsanguinator up the limb. A pneumatic tourniquet is then inflated around the thigh.

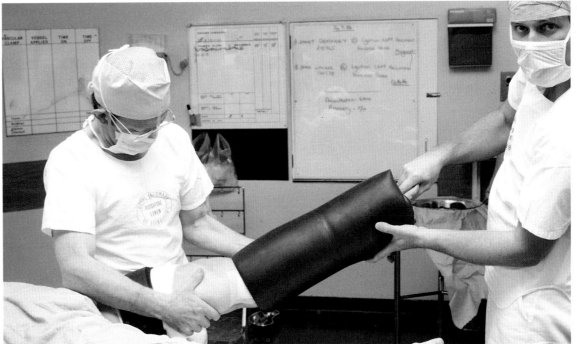

8 Recurrent Varicose Veins

This common problem can present considerable difficulties of assessment and dissection. It has to be acknowledged, and patients warned, that varices have a natural tendency to recur and that new sites of incompetence may develop. **All too often, however, recurrences are due to failure of pre-operative assessment or to inadequate surgery**[1].

Varicose veins can be divided into two types: residual and recurrent veins. RESIDUAL VARICES consist of gradually enlarging tortuous tributaries left behind after previous proximal incompetence has been dealt with. They can be treated by avulsion but usually sclerotherapy is all that is required. RECURRENT VARICES are fed by incompetent communications between the deep and superficial systems which were missed at the first operation or have become incompetent since. For these, further surgery is usually necessary.

1 and 2 In this patient the scars of the previous incisions have been highlighted to show the relationship with the recurrent varices. Clearly, there is still major deep to superficial reflux in the upper thigh.

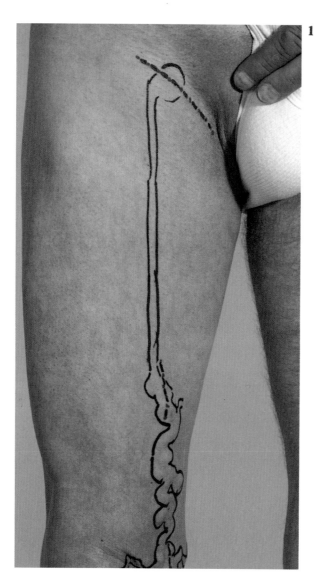
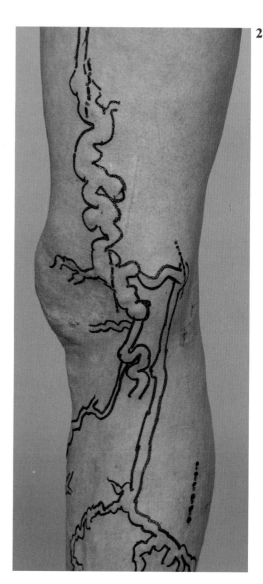

Investigation

Recurrent varices require thorough assessment. The possibility that the dilated superficial veins are acting as collaterals for obstructed deep veins must be excluded by careful history and, if in doubt, phlebography. The skin and subcutaneous tissues are often scarred and thickened by inflammation and oedema, so that clinical and Doppler examination are not so easy and may leave doubt as to the position of the incompetent communications.

Perforators can be detected by ascending phlebography (see page 25). It can be difficult to define recurrence at the saphenofemoral junction by either technique and descending phlebography is more effective at this level. Thus, close collaboration is essential between the surgeon and a radiologist who is specifically interested in the field.

3 Phlebographic studies are normally obtained pre-operatively but it is possible to obtain a varicogram on the table, if necessary.

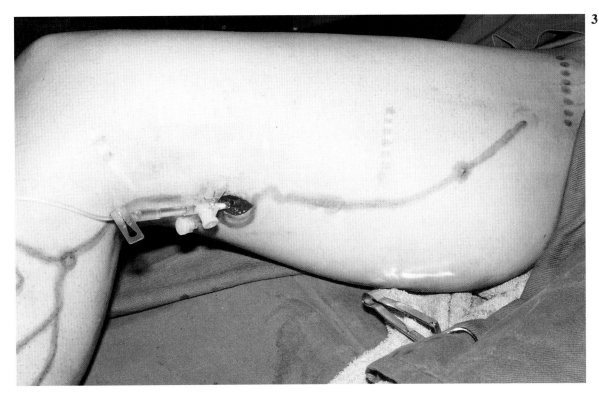

3

Re-exploration of the saphenofemoral junction

This operation should not be attempted by the unsupervised inexperienced surgeon. Usually multiple thin-walled veins are embedded in a mat of fibrous tissue overlying the saphenofemoral junction. Direct re-exploration of the junction by dissection through the scar can therefore be very difficult. It is only worth attempting if the previous incision has been placed so low as to suggest that by directing the dissection superiorly and preferably through a higher skin incision, satisfactory access to the junction can be obtained.

4 The scar of the previous operation has been dotted in. Multiple varices can be seen draining into the region of the saphenofemoral junction.

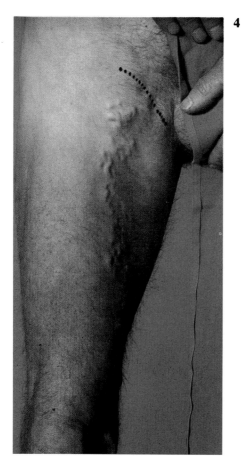

4

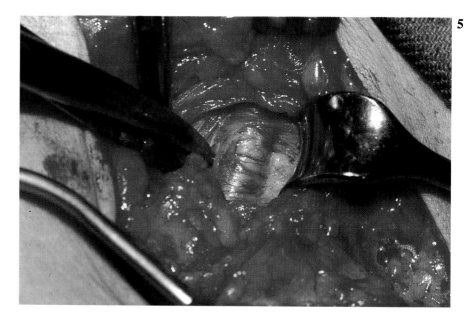

5

5 The recommended approach is to expose the vessels through an 'inverted hockey-stick' incision. This begins transversely just below the medial end of the inguinal ligament and turns down along the line of the femoral artery. The dissection is deepened to expose the common femoral artery.

6 The dissection is then carried medially to expose the common femoral vein and the long saphenous vein where it enters its anterior surface.

7 A sling has been placed around the upper end of the long saphenous vein to show it clearly where it emerges from the overlying scar tissue.

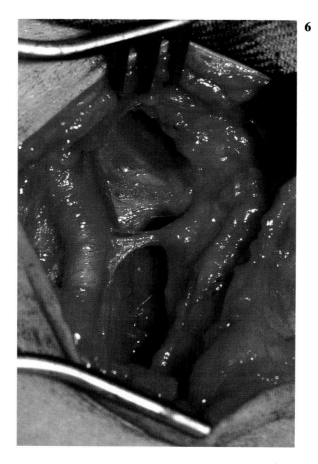

6

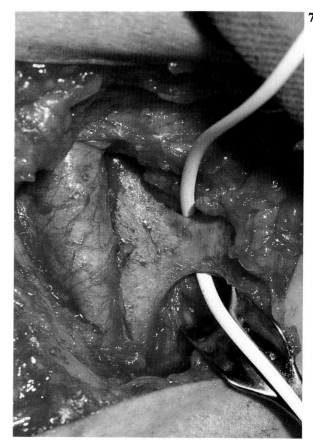

7

8 The saphenous vein is transfixed and ligated with non-absorbable suture.

9 A scalpel is being used to divide the saphenous vein. The stump can then be turned forwards to allow the junction and the adjacent common femoral vein to be searched for other tributaries such as the deep external pudendal vein, which should be divided.

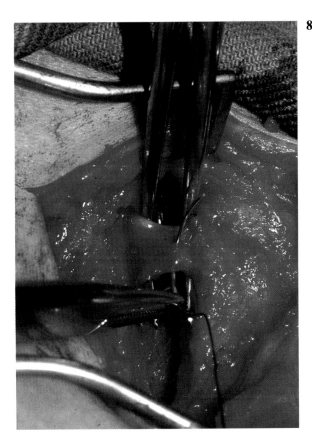
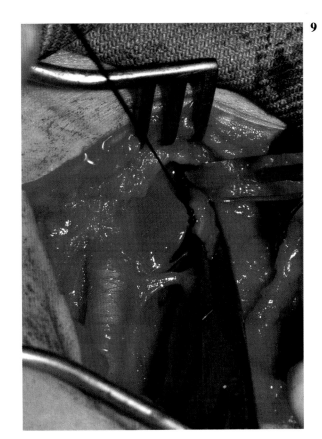

Division of the long saphenous vein alone is not sufficient to correct variceal recurrence. The next step in the operation is to dissect out the veins connected to the junction and also the distal long saphenous vein, if prior examination or phlebography has shown it to be present. There are two ways of proceeding.

10 The first alternative is to remove the overlying scar tissue and varices *en bloc*. This method has usually been adopted by the author. All vascular tissues, including lymphatics, entering the scar are serially ligated with synthetic absorbable ligatures and divided.

The yellow sling is around the femoral artery.

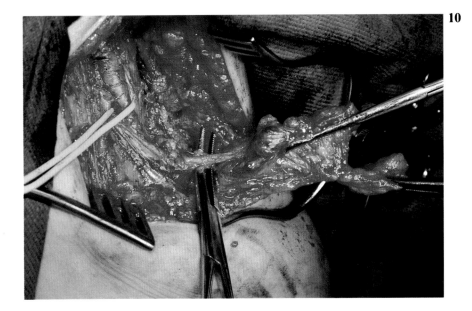

11 The area overlying the saphenofemoral junction has been cleared completely.

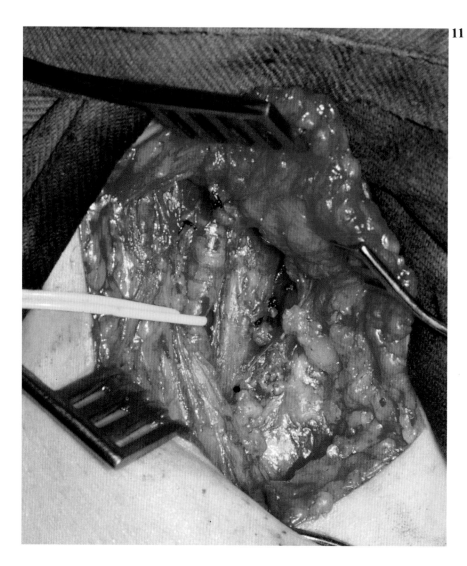

However, theoretically at least, this method may cause damage to lymphatic tissue and give rise to peripheral oedema or leakage of lymph from the wound.

An alternative to *en bloc* removal is to dissect around the perimeter of the scar tissue and individually intercept the veins draining into the area, after transfixing and dividing the saphenofemoral junction. The distal long saphenous is located at the lower border of the scar. It can be identified, if necessary, by passing a stripper up from a lower level **provided that one is aware of the danger that the stripper can occasionally pass into the femoral vein via a thigh perforator.**

Ligation or avulsion of distal perforators and varices, as described for primary varicose veins, completes the operation. The presence of scars or chronic inflammation in the lower leg mean that the operation is easier to perform under tourniquet.

9 Perivulval Varices

Varices in the pudendal region may stem from several possible sites of incompetence. These include the saphenofemoral junction via the superficial and deep external pudendal veins, the ovarian veins via the inguinal canal or the internal iliac veins via the obturator, internal pudendal or inferior gluteal veins. They develop during pregnancy and may largely or completely regress after delivery. **Surgery is never undertaken during pregnancy and is reserved for patients whose varices fail to regress spontaneously**[1]. Sclerotherapy is not effective.

Phlebography is advised in order to trace the source of the varices. Those stemming from saphenofemoral incomptence can be identified by ascending or descending phlebography and dealt with by juxtafemoral ligation, care being taken to ligate the deep external pudendal vein as well as the more superficial tributaries. Ovarian varices can be demonstrated by selective perfemoral catheterisation. Like scrotal varicocele, these can be dealt with by embolisation or by retroperitoneal ligations[2].

Veins draining from the pelvis can be intercepted through skin-crease incisions at the lateral edge of the vulva and at the lower edge of the buttock. **Care must be taken to dissect to a sufficient depth and to ligate or oversew all the veins crossing into the labium majus.** Veins coursing down the inner and posterior aspects of the thigh are removed by avulsion.

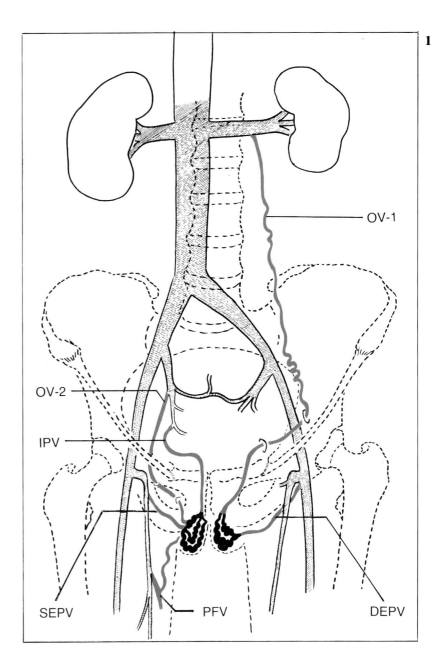

OV-1—ovarian vein
OV-2—obturator vein
IPV—internal pudendal vein
SEPV—superficial external pudendal vein
PFV—posteromedial femoral vein
DEPV—deep external pudendal vein

1 This composite diagram shows the principal channels draining the veins of the vulva. The superficial external pudendal vein drains into the upper end of the long saphenous vein or into the posteromedial femoral vein. The deep external pudendal vein joins the femoral vein at the saphenofemoral junction or it may join the long saphenous vein itself. Analogous to the varicocele in the male, vulval varices may be caused by distension of gonadal veins which pass from the vulva up the round ligament to the external inguinal ring, through the inguinal canal and up the posterior abdominal wall to join the left renal vein. More posteriorly the vulval veins drain into the internal iliac system via the obturator vein and the internal pudendal vein. It may be difficult or impossible to ascertain by physical examination which of these channels are important in an individual patient. Varicography is necessary, including selective catheterisation of the left gonadal vein via the left renal vein.

10 Venous Malformations

Vascular malformations are seen most commonly in the lower limbs. There is a slight preponderance of females. The most frequent symptoms are skin discoloration, pain and swelling. Congestive cardiac failure is a rare complication. Most present in childhood[1].

It is not always easy to be sure, when dealing with congenital venous malformations, whether or not arteriovenous fistula is present (Parkes-Weber syndrome), because limb lengthening and soft-tissue hypertrophy can occur in venous angioma without fistula.

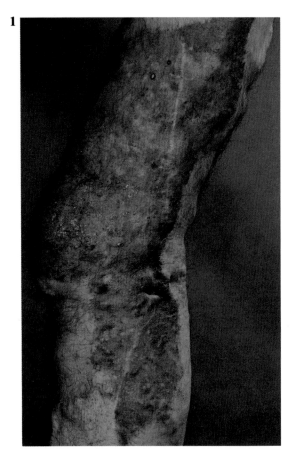 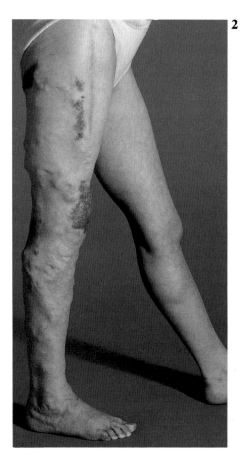 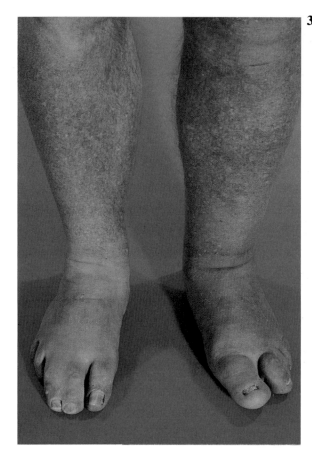

1 The combination of congenital varicose veins, cutaneous haemangiomas and overgrowth of the extremity with hypertrophy of soft tissue and bone, was described by Klippel and Trenaunay in 1900[2].

2 The varices are typically situated posterolaterally.

3 In addition to overgrowth of soft tissues, this patient has congenital fusion of toes.

4 In mild forms the Klippel-Trenaunay syndrome presents as atypical posterolateral varices with barely visible capillary haemangioma.

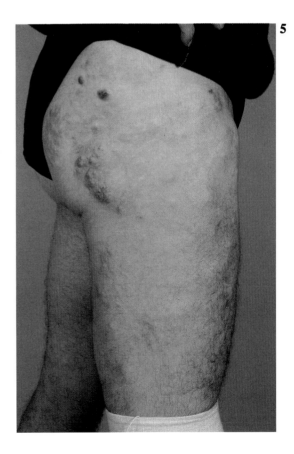

Arteriovenous fistula

Arteriovenous fistulas, because of their more serious prognosis, if possible require active intervention. Major fistulas can be treated by direct surgical attack with ligation of the feeding arteries. Usually, however, this is technically not possible either because of inaccessibility or because of the danger of devitalising large areas of tissue. Embolisation by selective catheterisation of the feeding vessels, usually done as staged treatment, has opened up a new and often highly successful mode of treatment.

Caution: Ligation of feeding arteries should never be undertaken without careful consideration and discussion with the radiologist because it will prevent subsequent catheter access. The same applies to attempts to control haemorrhage by arterial ligature.

5 The hemi pelvis is a common site for congenital AV fistula, which may present in the buttock or upper thigh. Auscultation may reveal the classical machinery murmur of a sizeable fistula but generally congenital fistulas are small, diffuse and multiple. The presence of arteriovenous shunting is inferred from the clinical features. The actual arteriovenous connections cannot be demonstrated readily by conventional arteriography. This is one of the areas where Digital subtraction angiography offers advantages.

6 This girl has considerable lengthening of the right leg as a result of congenital AV fistula. Limb overgrowth was formerly treated by epiphyseal stapling, but now it is regarded as preferable to wait until growth is complete and then to carry out a formal limb shortening operation.

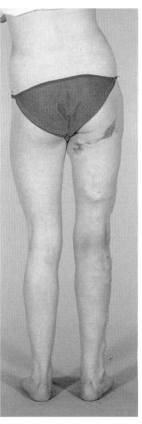

Phlebangioma

This collective term includes a variety of localised congenital malformations or hamartomas. In addition to occurring in the Klippel-Trenaunay syndrome in association with varicose veins and limb overgrowth, they may exist separately as surface capillary haemangiomas (as shown here) or more deeply placed cavernous haemangiomas.

The mainstay of treatment for this condition when it occurs in the lower limb is graduated elastic compression (page 114). This will protect the patient from progression of the condition and from the skin consequences of chronic venous hypertension.

Surgery should be avoided as a rule. Rarely it may have a place in reducing bulky varicosities and ameliorating cutaneous capillary haemangiomas if they are bleeding or are particularly unsightly, as was the case illustrated. The role of laser therapy still has to be defined.

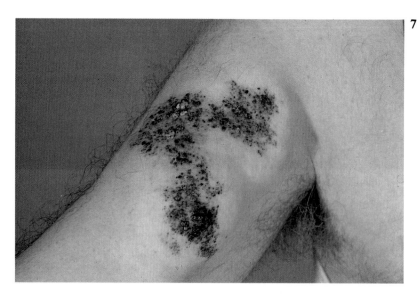

7 This angioma was treated by radical excision and skin-grafting. Before undertaking excision of superficial veins in this group of conditions, the patency of the deep veins should be confirmed by phlebography.

Incisions over haemangiomatous areas of skin are to be avoided, because they tend to break down and lead to chronic ulceration.

Angiosarcoma

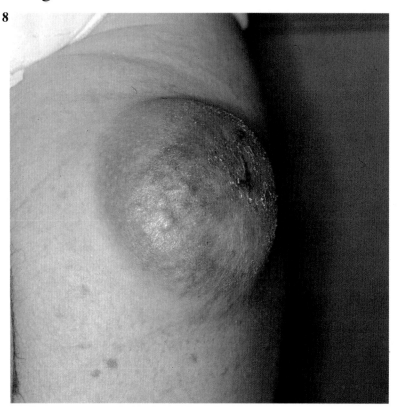

8 This patient had a small capillary angioma of the buttock, first noticed in childhood. It remained quiescent until she became pregnant, when rapid enlargement occurred.

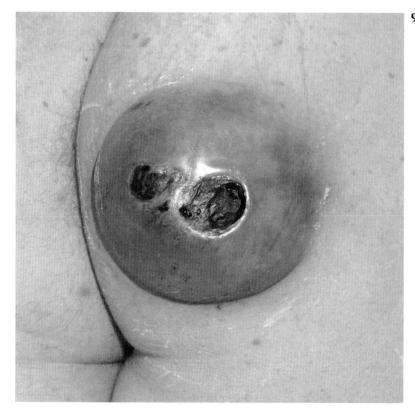

9 Breakdown of the overlying skin resulted in severe bleeding.

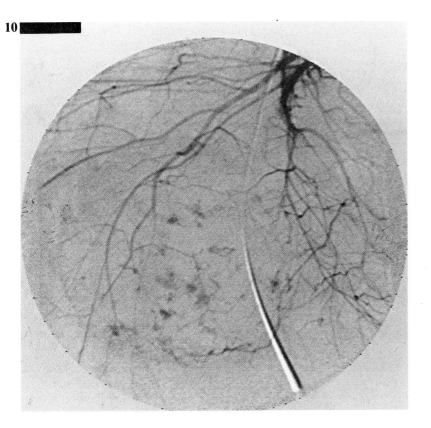

10 Digital subtraction angiography showed a well circumscribed lesion with multiple microvascular AV connections. The lesion was treated by embolisation of the relevant branches of the inferior gluteal and internal pudendal arteries.

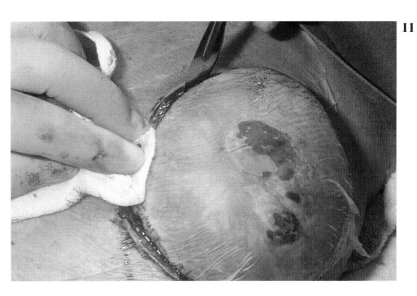

11 This resulted in shrinkage of the mass. On the day after the embolisation it was excised through a circumferential incision. A plastic dressing was applied to the surface to seal the ulcerated area.

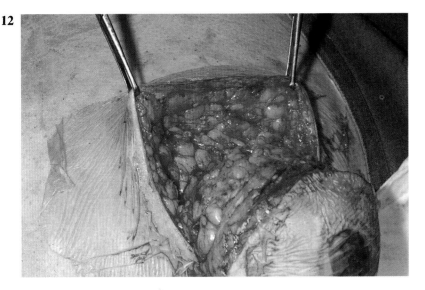

12 The embolisation having effectively thrombosed the tumour, it could be excised *en bloc* with a generous margin of normal tissue. There was only minor bleeding.

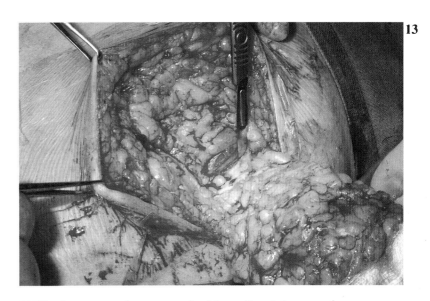

13 The deepest portion was excised from the gluteus maximus.

14

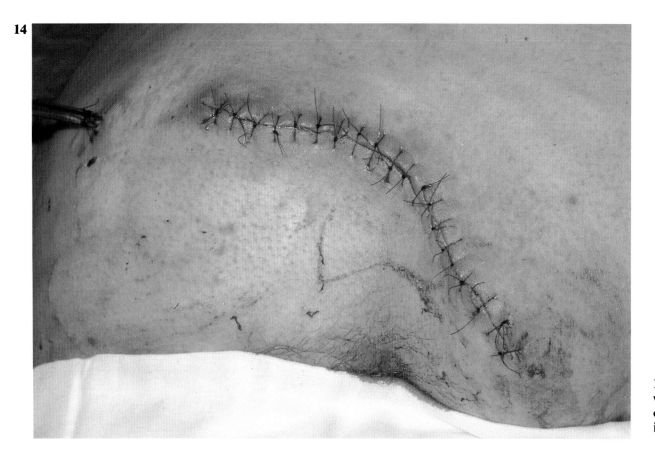

14 The defect was closed over a wide-bore vacuum drain, brought out through a stab-wound incision.

15

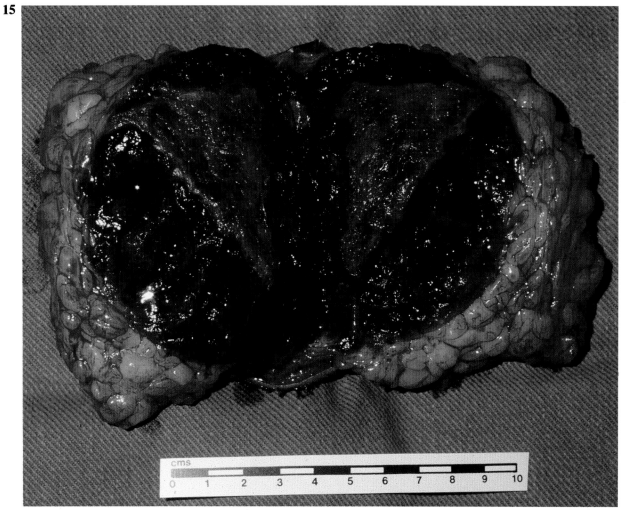

15 The transected specimen showed that it had been infarcted by the embolisation. Histological examination showed the tumour to be an angiosarcoma which was reported by the pathologist to have been completely excised locally. Sadly, however, a few months later widespread bony metastases appeared.

11 Venous Thrombosis and Pulmonary Embolism

Venous thrombo-embolism is in the main a benign and self-limiting disease. Consequently most patients survive, thus perpetuating polices of investigation and treatment which are often inadequate for that minority of patients who are seriously affected. It is important for the clinician to be alert to the situations in which it is necessary to apply an approach that is different from routine conventional courses of heparin and oral anticoagulants.

The aims of management are as follows:
1 To facilitate resolution of the acute episode.
2 To avert major pulmonary embolism.
3 To prevent recurrence.
4 To minimise post-thrombotic sequelae.

Diagnosis

It cannot be overemphasised that the key to treatment is accurate diagnosis. So unreliable is the clinical diagnosis of deep vein thrombosis (DVT) and of pulmonary embolism that additional investigation is required if the full aims of treatment, as listed above, are to be realised. **Anticoagulants are dangerous drugs, responsible for a great deal of morbidity and occasional deaths**[1]. Precise diagnosis is advocated not only to enable treatment to be tailored to the nature and severity of thrombo-embolism, but also to allow anticoagulants and other treatments to be safely withheld or reduced to a minimum. Although a variety of methods of diagnosing DVT have been advocated, phlebography is still unsurpassed.

In some hospitals a screening service is available using strain gauge or electrical impedance plethysmography, thermography or duplex imaging. These techniques, if performed by an experienced doctor or technician, are useful in that they may lessen the pressure on the radiology department and reduce the number of negative phlebograms.

Phlebography remains the crucial investigation in the management of both DVT and pulmonary embolism. It not only clarifies the diagnosis but also, by defining the site, extent and nature of the thrombus, in a way that the above screening tests cannot do, makes a selective policy of management possible.

The exception to this is the patient who presents with MASSIVE LIFE-THREATENING EMBOLISM when attention must obviously be focused on the heart and lungs. Bedside echo-cardiography can be helpful while resuscitation is proceeding and urgent pulmonary angiography is being arranged. **Lung scanning in these circumstances wastes valuable time.** If, as is usual, thrombolytic therapy is chosen as the treatment for massive embolism, it becomes less important to carry out phlebography because the source thrombus is also being treated. But if the patient fails to respond to medical treatment, and pulmonary embolectomy is employed, further embolism remains a threat, so a phlebogram should then be considered as a preliminary to the placement of a caval filter.

When a patient presents with a clinical diagnosis of PULMONARY EMBOLISM WHICH IS LESS THAN 'LIFE-THREATENING', the urgent priority is to find out whether potentially lethal thrombus is present in the peripheral veins. This usually means the veins of the lower limbs and pelvis, because embolism from the veins of the upper limbs is relatively uncommon. The reason for this approach is that the majority of fatal emboli are preceded by smaller 'herald' emboli[2-4].

For 'sub-massive' emboli a perfusion lung scan is a reasonable alternative to pulmonary angiography. The limitations of lung scanning have to be understood. A clearly positive or a clearly negative lung scan is a valuable aid to clinical management. However, there is quite a large intermediate group of scans which show minor perfusion defects and which have to be interpreted with caution in the light of other evidence. However, they can still be valuable as baseline investigations. The addition of ventilation scanning improves the accuracy slightly, but only in patients with large perfusion defects[5].

If the patient presents with SUSPECTED DVT, the objective is the same (that is to exclude potentially lethal thrombus). A further objective is to minimise the damaging sequelae of DVT in the limb. The critical investigation, on both counts, is a phlebogram (refer to page 24).

It is important to consider carefully the type of phlebogram required (page 26). The aim of the examination is not merely to confirm the diagnosis but also to define the thrombus accurately, especially its upper extent because this is the dangerous portion. Close liaison between surgeon and radiologist is essential so that the correct type of phlebogram may be chosen, taking into account the clinical presentation. For example, if there is swelling in the thigh, ascending phlebography is unlikely to give satisfactory delineation of the pelvic part of the thrombus.

In suspected embolism and also in DVT the phlebogram should be bilateral even though the symptoms may only be on one side. The reasons are that silent but clinically important thrombus may often be revealed and secondly the simultaneous flow of contrast up both legs is generally necessary to give adequate definition of pelvic veins and cava.

When a patient presents with symptoms of DVT we believe it is also important at an early stage, regardless of whether or not the patient has any chest symptoms, to obtain a PERFUSION LUNG SCAN, partly because it very often reveals unsuspected embolism and partly because it provides a valuable baseline against which to measure future events.

The clinical features of deep vein thrombosis

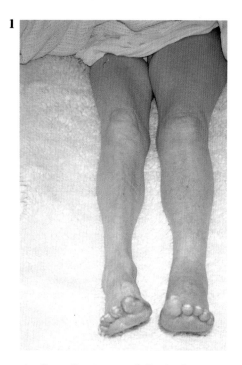

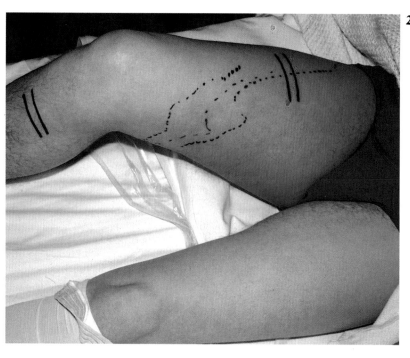

1 Deep vein thrombosis is most often silent, especially in its early stages. A swelling, such as this, means extensive thrombus with a substantial degree of outflow obstruction.

2 The swollen leg is generally pale (phlegmasia alba dolens). However, some patients with DVT show an unusually active inflammatory response to the thrombus, evident as tenderness and erythema in the groin.

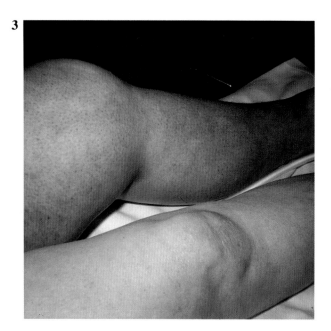

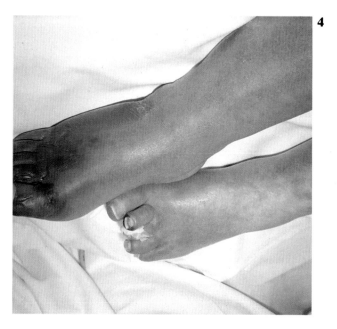

3 Phlegmasia caerulea dolens indicates a severe degree of obstruction to venous outflow occasioned by thrombosis not only of main channels but also of collaterals. Large amounts of body fluid can be sequestered in the limb, resulting in serious fluid and electrolyte disturbance. **The rise in tissue pressure may cause arterial obstruction leading to gangrene.**

4 Venous gangrene. This condition is, fortunately, relatively rare. In the author's experience it is usually associated with advanced malignant disease. The limb is grossly swollen with blistering. **Despite the alarming appearances the surgeon should not be tempted to carry out limb amputation at an early stage.** Excisional surgery should be deferred until swelling and venous return have been ameliorated by all possible means. Excision can then usually be extremely conservative, preserving all but frankly necrotic tissue.

Treatment

In so far as it is possible to generalise in a diverse condition standard care is as follows.

If the patient presents with suspected DVT or an embolism which is not life-threatening, heparin therapy is started promptly while awaiting phlebography (subject to the comments on screening tests in the section on diagnosis) and a perfusion lung scan. These should be performed within 24 hours. Heparin treatment is started by bolus intravenous injection followed by continuous infusion. The patient is nursed with the foot of the bed elevated and, if there is leg swelling, extra elevation of the affected limb should be obtained. Ankle exercises are encouraged. **No attempt is made to reduce swelling by means of elastic compression which can do more harm than good in this situation.** Compression is not applied until the patient starts to walk.

The heparin therapy is given as an intravenous loading dose of 5,000-10,000 u, depending on the size and age of the patient and the severity of the event, followed by 1,500-3,000 u per hour by infusion pump.

The dose should be controlled with care by monitoring the activated partial thromboplastin time aiming at two to two-and-a-half times the control value. Monitoring is especially important over the first few days because heparin requirements vary considerably and surprisingly large doses may be needed in the presence of a new and extensive thrombus. Heparin is continued for a week or longer if the thrombosis is a large one.

Twice daily subcutaneous injections of calcium heparin are an effective alternative to intravenous heparin[6]. The initial treatment is 2,500 u per 10 kg body weight, given every 12 hours. Subsequent doses are adjusted to maintain a coagulation time approximately twice that of control.

The heparin is overlapped with warfarin by 3-4 days. The conventional overlap period of 48 hours is insufficient for an oral anticoagulant to achieve its full effect and relapse can occur at the transition stage.

The patient starts to mobilise with elastic support after 48 hours of heparin therapy, provided the swelling has been controlled. Warfarin is continued for three months; longer, if there are post-thrombotic symptoms or a history of recurrent episodes.

High quality graduated compression stockings are prescribed for as long as post-thrombotic symptoms persist.

Thrombolytic therapy

Thrombolytic therapy has recently entered a new phase with the emergence of new agents: anisoylated plasminogen-streptokinase complex (APSAC), recombinant tissue plasminogen activator and pro-urokinase[7]. These agents have greater fibrin specificity and appear to carry less risk of causing bleeding complications. The extent to which they are superior to streptokinase and urokinase is not yet clear.

If the patient presents with massive pulmonary embolism, the emergency measures include oxygen, 15,000 u of heparin and, if necessary, cardiac massage. If the patient is failing to maintain systemic blood pressure, intravenous fluids must be infused to support right ventricular output. Through a separate drip a vasoconstrictor is given. Noradrenaline is made up as 2 mg in 500 ml of isotonic saline and administered through a paediatric burette which allows the dose to be titrated accurately to give the required blood pressure of at least 80 mmHg systolic. Should there be delay in obtaining pulmonary angiography and the patient's condition warrants it, thrombolytic therapy can be given at this stage. Our preference, however, is to obtain angiography first. **If this confirms the diagnosis and the patient's condition remains serious, thrombolytic therapy is given immediately, either via the angiogram catheter or via a peripheral line.**

Streptokinase is given as a loading dose of 250,000 u followed by 100,000 u per hour for 24 hours. APSAC can be given as a single intravascular bolus while rt-PA is given as a loading dose followed by a maintenance infusion. These new agents are still being evaluated in the treatment of pulmonary embolism; the advice of the manufacturer should be sought over their administration and monitoring. The duration of thrombolytic therapy depends on the clinical and radiological response. Pulmonary embolectomy is required very rarely.

The results of lytic therapy for lower limb DVT have in general been disappointing, both in terms of the early success rate and the avoidance of post-thrombotic sequelae[8-10]. Thus, as far as streptokinase and urokinase are concerned, their use does not seem to be justified in the light of sometimes serious side effects and of costs. It remains to be seen whether the new agents have anything more to offer.

A more optimistic view of lytic therapy can be taken with upper limb and superior caval thrombosis. A tendency to give rise to symptoms at an earlier stage appears to make these thrombi more susceptible to lysis[11] (see page 80). Remember that subclavian vein thrombosis may be a manifestation of thoracic outlet compression requiring operative correction[12,13].

Venous thrombectomy in the lower limb

Venous thrombectomy is less popular than formerly. It incurs appreciable morbidity and thrombectomised veins have a strong tendency to re-thrombose, especially on the left side. However, good results have recently been reported both in terms of early success and of long-term avoidance of post-phlebitic sequelae[14,15]. These authors have combined their thrombectomy with the construction of an arteriovenous fistula which is probably essential if the thrombectomised vein is to remain patent.

Indications

For thrombectomy to be worth considering the onset of the DVT, as judged by the clinical circumstances and the radiological appearances, must be recent (that is within the previous week). The thrombus has usually been present much longer than the symptoms, often by many days or even weeks. There is no point in considering thrombectomy if the precipitating cause, such as pelvic sepsis or tumour, is still present. The patient must be capable of mobilising after operation and of using the muscles and joints of the lower limbs effectively. Thrombectomy is usually performed only for high segment DVT and the right side has a better prospect of remaining patent than the left. Some surgeons now regard the only indication for thrombectomy to be limb-threatening phlegmasia caerulea dolens.

The operation

The operation is performed under general anaesthesia with continuous positive pressure ventilation. The patient is supine and the table in the reversed Trendelenburg position. Intravenous heparin is continued throughout. It is an advantage, but not essential, to have an image intensifier in theatre.

5a and b These phlebo-grams show a right iliofemoral DVT which is non-occlusive in the thigh but is occluding the right external and common iliac veins completely. This condition was successfully treated by thrombectomy.

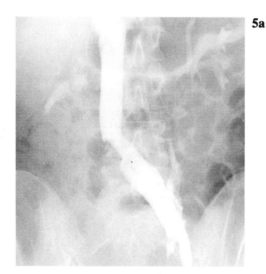

5a

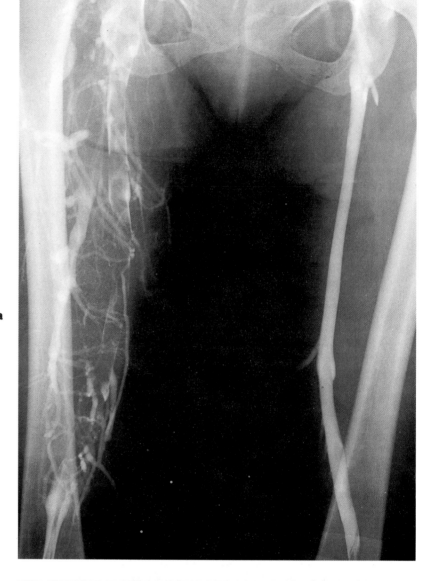

5b

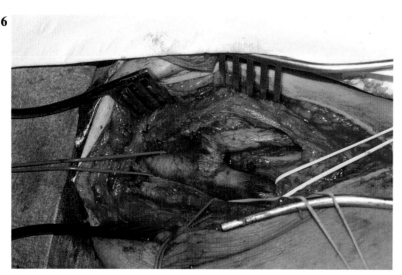

6

6 The common femoral artery and vein are exposed through a longitudinal incision. The femoral vein can be seen to be bulging with thrombus. Plastic slings are applied. Care is taken not to compress the veins at this stage.

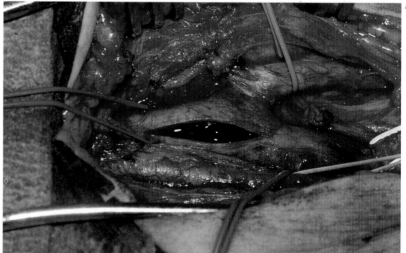

7

7 A venotomy is made and thrombus allowed to bulge out. If the vein is of narrow calibre, a transverse venotomy is preferred.

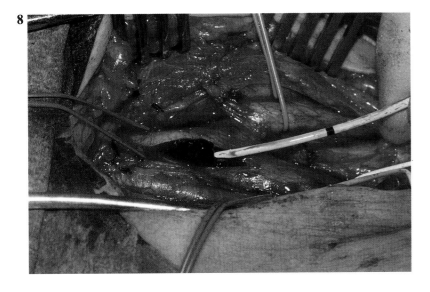

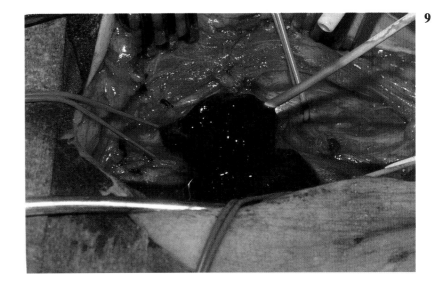

8 While the anaesthetist maintains positive pressure a Fogarty catheter is passed up through the thrombus. If the operation is being done on the left side, the image intensifier may be used to check that the catheter has not entered the ascending lumbar vein.

9 The balloon is inflated and the thrombus withdrawn.

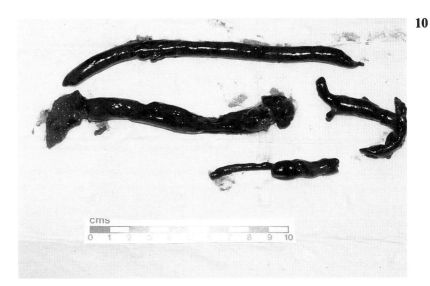

10 The removed thrombus. At its point of origin the primary thrombus is pale, adherent and difficult to extract. The great bulk of the material is secondary or propagated thrombus which, provided the onset is recent, is easy to remove.

11 With the leg raised and the proximal common femoral vein clamped, thrombus is manually expressed from the veins of the calf and thigh. Here the surgeon is running his thumbs with firm pressure along the course of the femoral vein in the thigh. The expressed thrombus is being picked up with forceps. An Esmarch bandage can also be used to expel distal thrombus.

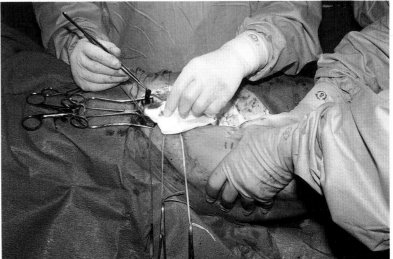

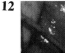12

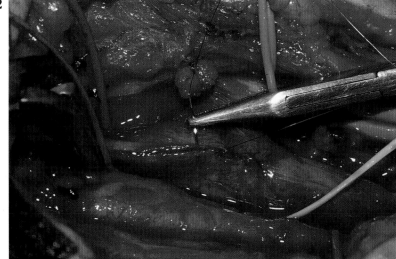

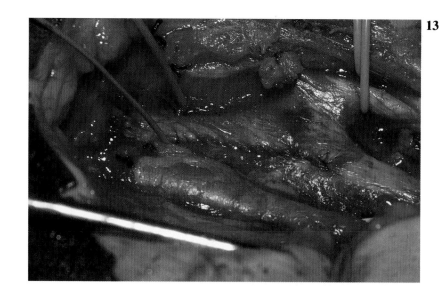13

12 The venotomy is closed with a fine monofilament suture.

13 The closed venotomy.

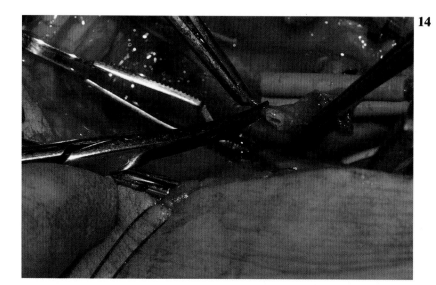14

14 To fashion an arteriovenous fistula the long saphenous vein is divided about 6 cm below the saphenofemoral junction and turned laterally to be anastomosed to the femoral artery. If there is any back bleeding, it is clamped gently with a rubber-shod bulldog. Here, the adventitia is being cleaned away before anastomosis.

As an alternative to making the fistula with the saphenous vein itself, a large tributary can be used.

15 The back row of the end-to-side anastomosis between saphenous vein and femoral artery has been completed as a purse-string.

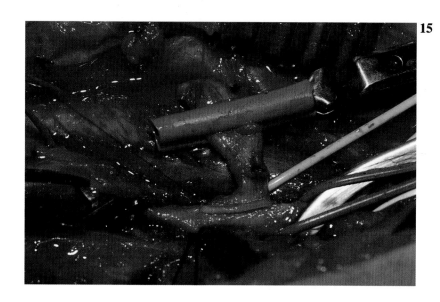15

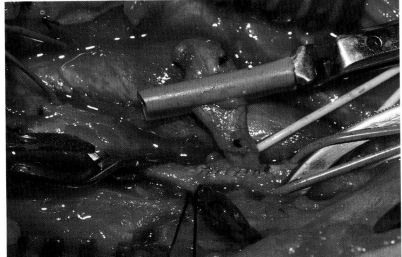

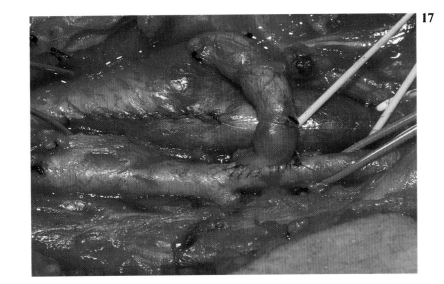

16 The front row is now complete.

17 The clamp is removed and the fistula distends.

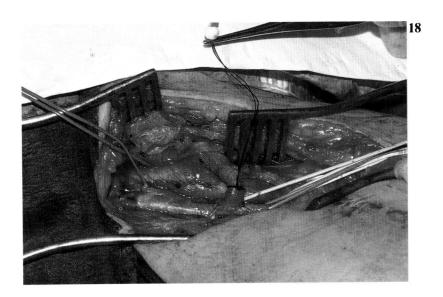

18 To facilitate later closure of the AV fistula, a non-absorbable ligature is placed around the fistula and secured with a bead just under the skin. A fine catheter is tied into one of the tributaries of the long saphenous vein and brought out through a stab incision, so that phlebography can be carried out 2-4 days later to check its patency.

Aftercare

The patient is nursed with the leg well elevated for 3-4 days and is maintained on intravenous heparin for 10 days overlapped for 4 days with oral anticoagulant (warfarin), which is continued for at least 6 months. When walking commences a graduated compression stocking is applied. The arteriovenous fistula is closed 6 weeks later.

Caval interruption

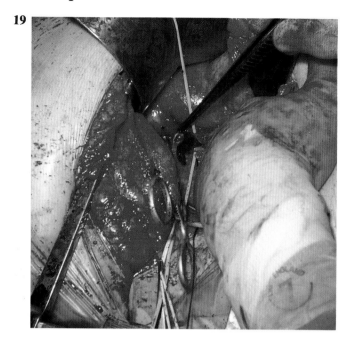

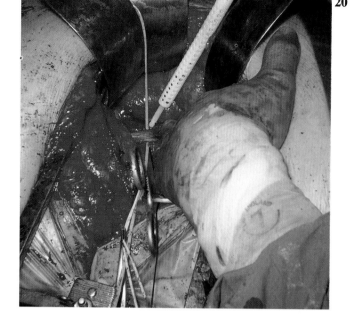

Direct caval interruption by ligature, suture or clip has largely been replaced by transvenous filter techniques. However, if an intra-abdominal operation is being performed for other reasons in a patient known to be at high risk of thrombo-embolism, it is a relatively simple and potentially life-saving matter to apply a serrated (Miles) clip to the inferior vena cava[16].

19 The cava may be approached extraperitoneally or transperitoneally. This patient had an extensive caval and iliac thrombosis and thrombectomy was performed before the application of a clip. An extraperitoneal approach was used through a transverse subcostal incision, and the cava exposed just below the liver. A sling was placed gently around the cava. Because the thrombus extended up to the diaphragm, a clamp was not applied until the cava had been opened and the proximal tongue of thrombus extracted by Fogarty catheter. The thrombus can be seen extruding. A soft-jaw clamp was then applied across the cava above the thrombus.

20 Distal thrombus has been extracted by suction and by thrombectomy catheter. The venotomy is ready for closure with fine monofilament.

21 The Miles clip. A silk ligature has been placed through the hole in the clip ready for tying once it is in position.

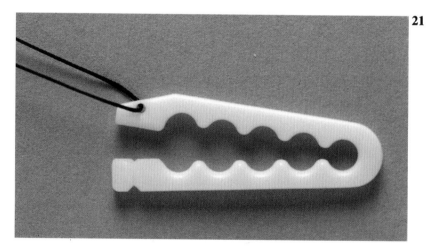

22 Here the clip is being held in forceps before being put into position.
This is done by passing the right-angled forceps behind the cava, grasping the lower blade of the clip and drawing it through. The ligature is then tied to clamp it in position.

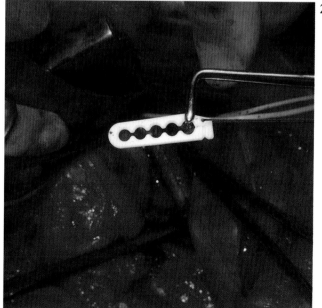

23 In this patient a transperitoneal approach was made and the duodenum reflected medially to give wide exposure of the cava. Note the clip in place.

Aftercare is similar to that described for thrombectomy.

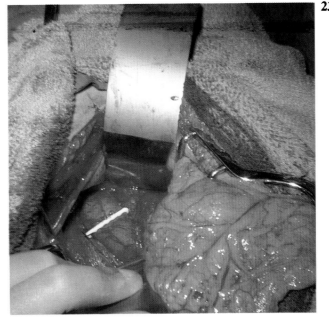

23

Inferior vena caval filters

The placement of a caval filter is most commonly indicated in patients who cannot be treated by anticoagulants or who suffer from embolism despite anticoagulation. It has also been our practice to insert a filter if a patient presenting with embolism or DVT is shown by phlebography to have potentially lethal thrombus. This usually means fresh thrombus extending proximal to the femoral vein, but clearly **if a patient already has limited respiratory function due to embolism or other lung disease, then even a small peripheral thrombus could be potentially lethal.** Hence the need for high quality phlebography which properly defines the thrombus.

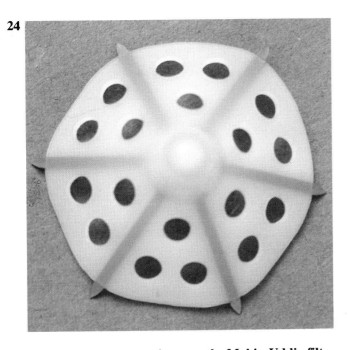

24 A popular early variety was the Mobin-Uddin filter.

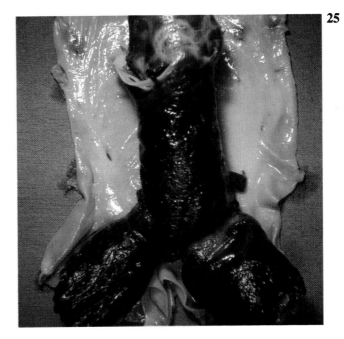

25 This type of filter tended to induce complete occlusion of the cava and thus aggravate post-thrombotic symptoms. This necropsy specimen shows thrombus below and above the filter. The Greenfield filter, the insertion of which is shown in the following series of photographs, is superior in this respect[17,18].

The insertion of a Greenfield filter

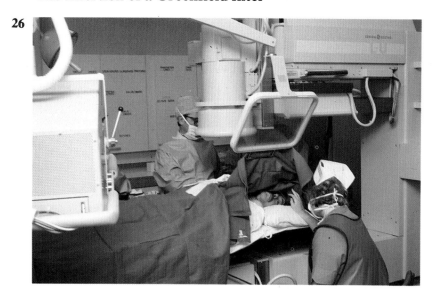

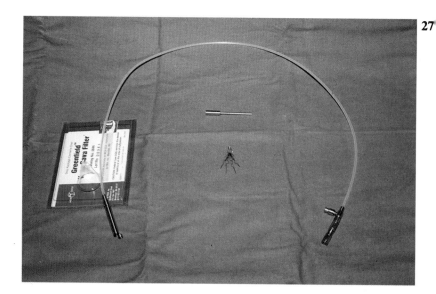

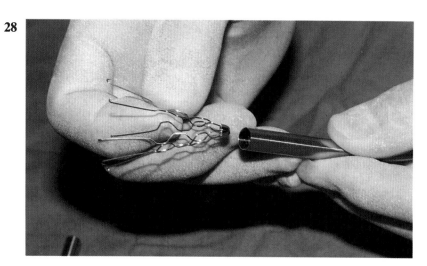

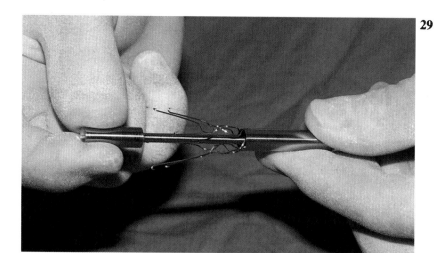

26 The operation is done under local anaesthesia with radiological control. The patient lies supine on the xray table with the head turned to the left. A nurse sits alongside for reassurance.

27 The filter and carrier are checked.

28 The filter is loaded into the carrier.

29 It is pushed into the carrying cylinder with a special tool.

30 The position is checked to ensure that the legs of the filter are not crossed.

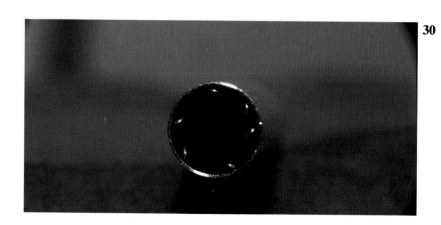

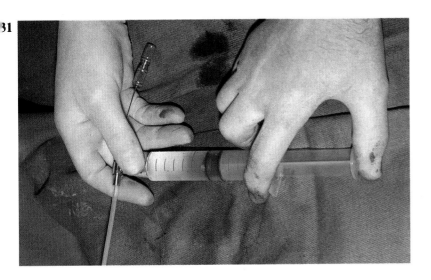

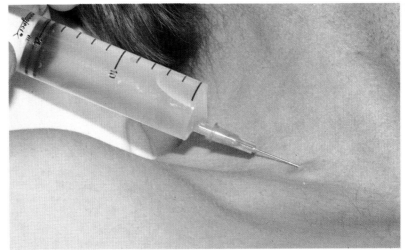

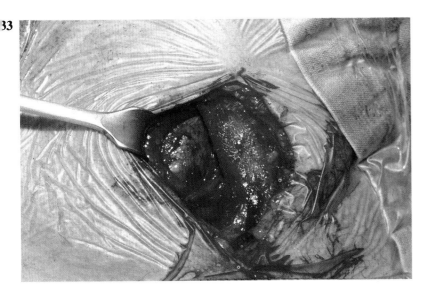

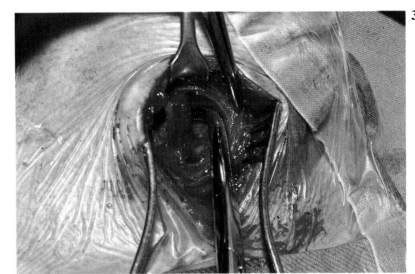

31 The whole system is then preloaded with heparinised saline.

32 The skin above the medial end of the clavicle is infiltrated with 1 per cent lignocaine.

33 Through a longitudinal incision, the 'V' between the sternal and clavicular heads of the sternomastoid muscle is exposed. The internal jugular vein lies immediately behind the 'V'.

34 Care must be taken in mobilising the vein, which is usually adherent to cervical fascia posteriorly. Here a dissecting forcep is being passed around the internal jugular vein.

35 A sling is placed around the vein.

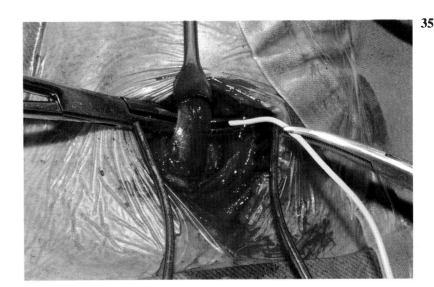

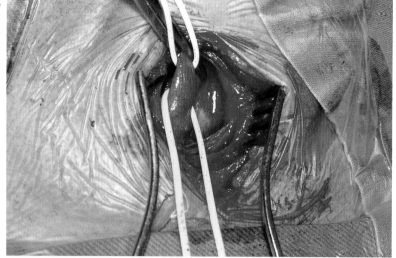

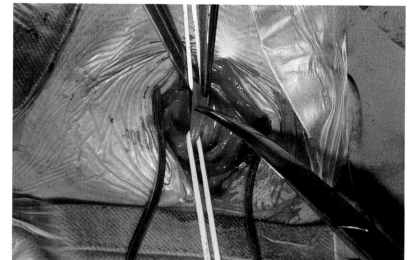

36 A second sling is applied above.

37 A transverse venotomy is made.

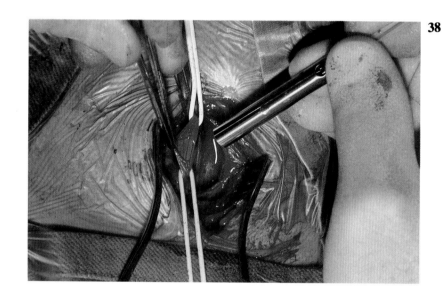

38 Care must be taken when introducing the carrier not to allow air embolism.

39 The carrier is passed down into the infrarenal inferior vena cava under radiological control. To negotiate past the heart and the right renal vein, it is sometimes necessary to rotate the patient on to the left side.

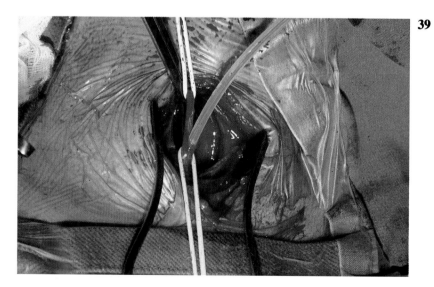

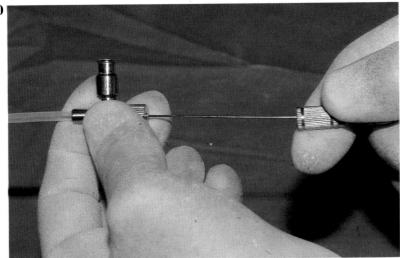

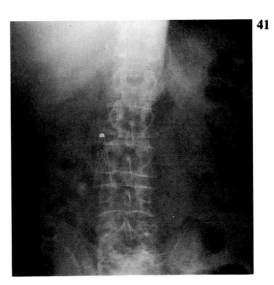

39

40 The position of the kidneys having previously been checked by the intravenous injection of contrast medium, the filter is released in the infrarenal cava. This is done by withdrawing the outer sleeve clear of the filter while holding steady the inner wire of the filter carrier. **Care should be taken not to release the filter in the right renal vein or the right common iliac vein.** After removal of the carrier, the venotomy in the internal jugular is closed with fine monofilament, or the vein can be ligated.

41 This film shows the filter in position.

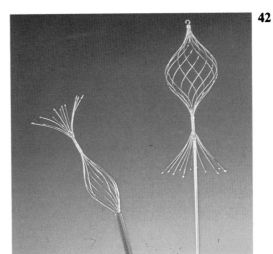

42 A recent further improvement is the development of methods of transvenous percutaneous filter insertion. This can be achieved via the groin or the neck. The Gunther filter[19], shown here, or the bird's-nest filter[20] may be used.

43 A post-insertion radiograph shows a Gunther filter in place.

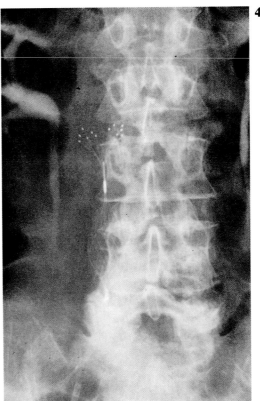

12 Venous Obstruction in the Upper Limb and Superior Vena Cava

Venous obstruction affecting the upper limb and/or superior mediastinum is relatively uncommon. Two varieties are recognised: acute thrombosis and chronic recurrent obstruction.

Acute thrombosis

There are primary and secondary types. Primary thrombosis occurs in otherwise healthy individuals, predominantly male, and often follows physical activity involving unusual straining or positioning of the limb—so-called 'effort' thrombosis. The term 'primary' is misleading because there is usually an underlying anatomical abnormality such as anomalous scalene bands or insufficient space between the clavicle and the first rib (page 17).

Secondary thrombosis of axillary and subclavian veins and cava may follow intravenous catheterisation, drug injection, neoplasm or trauma.

The signs and symptoms usually occur within 1 or 2 days of the precipitating event. They include swelling, venous engorgement and uncomfortable heaviness of the limb. In severe cases there may be numbness and parasthesiae. There may also be venous distension in the pectoral region. In secondary thrombosis there may, in addition, be the signs and symptoms of superior vena caval occlusion with swelling and venous engorgement of head and neck. The diagnosis is confirmed by phlebography.

Treatment

Anticoagulation and high elevation of the arm on pillows is the standard conservative treatment. Heparin is begun with an intravenous loading dose of 5,000-10,000 u followed by continuous infusion at a level to keep the activated partial thromboplastin time at approximately two to two-and-a-half times normal. This is continued for 7-10 days and overlapped with warfarin by 3-4 days.

Conservative treatment is the policy which is most widely practised, but recently authors have pointed out that it is followed by residual symptoms of pain, tiredness and parasthesiae in between 60 and 85 per cent of patients[1-4]. Many surgeons therefore take a more active approach using thrombolytic therapy, surgery or a combination of the two.

Because the acute symptoms tend to appear early, unlike DVT of the lower limb, thrombosis of the upper limb responds well to thrombolytic therapy, provided that it is started promptly[5,6].

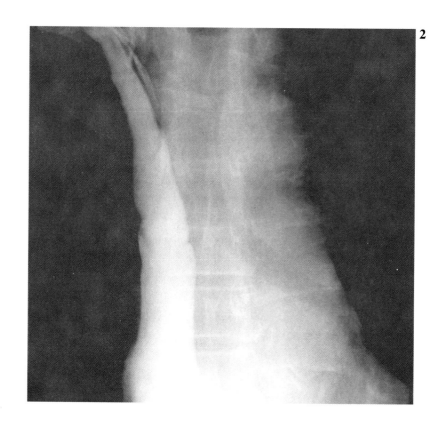

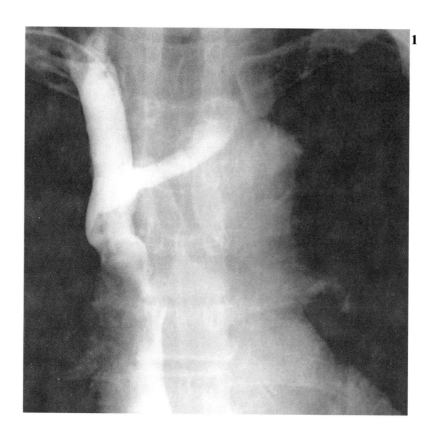

1 Phlebography showing thrombosis of the superior vena cava induced by a parenteral nutrition catheter, which is still in place.

2 Clearance of the cava effected by a single bolus of anisoylated plasminogen streptokinase (APSAC) via the catheter.

3 Effort thrombosis. Caused in this 60-year-old woman, who worked in a library, by repeatedly lifting heavy books from high shelves.

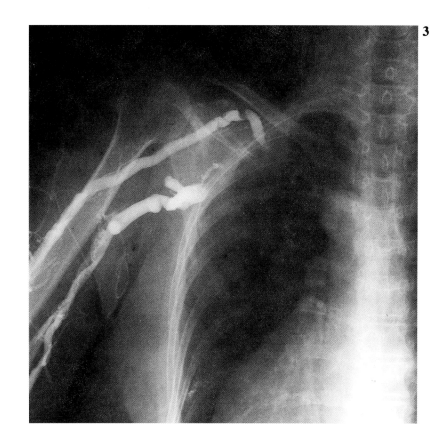

4 Clearance was achieved within 24 hours by two intravenous boluses of APSAC. The residual kink in the subclavian vein can be seen where it crosses the first rib. Recurrence of thrombosis is likely, unless the cause of compression is removed.

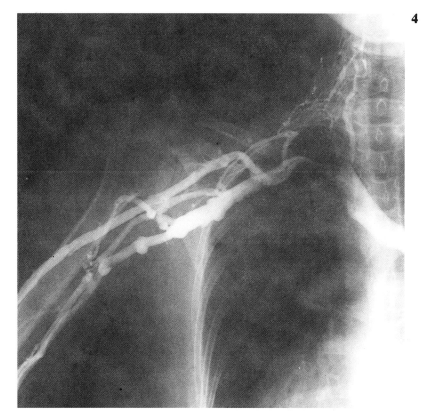

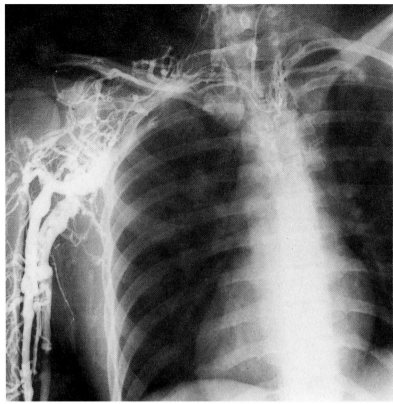

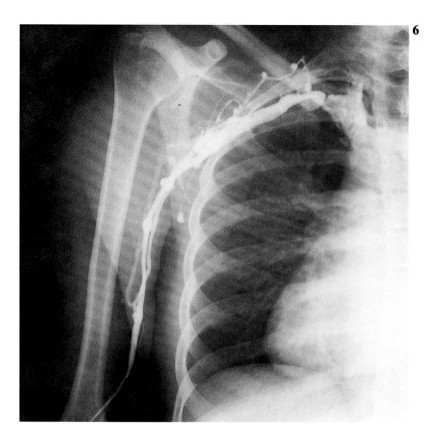

5 This recurrent axillary vein thrombosis, in a female ballet dancer, was caused by being repeatedly lifted up by the armpits by her dancing partner. Note the numerous collaterals.

6 After 2 days of thrombolytic therapy, the thrombus was completely cleared leaving a tight constriction clearly visible in the subclavian vein. Recurrence is therefore likely as long as the underlying mechanical defect remains.

Thombectomy has been advocated by a number of authors[7-9] with satisfactory long-term patency rates.

In the case of primary thrombosis, thrombectomy should be accompanied by measures to relieve the compression on the subclavian vein, such as first rib resection. Otherwise re-thrombosis will occur.

The same principle applies to thrombolytic therapy. Clearance of the thrombus should be followed by phlebographic studies to ascertain the presence of outlet compression which, depending on the circumstances of the patient, might be treated properly by operation. Although in some patients scalenotomy or division of fibrous bands appears to suffice, first rib resection is probably the most reliable procedure[10]. Thrombectomy can be done by the same route.

Chronic intermittent obstruction

This condition is uncommon and may occur with or without a history of venous thrombosis. The symptoms arise with various activities or positions of the arm. They are similar to those described for acute venous thrombosis but they are relieved by returning the limb to a relaxed position. The right arm is more frequently involved.

The symptoms can be reproduced by asking the patient to adopt the military position or by hyperabduction of the arm. Simultaneous venous pressure measurements show abnormal pressure rises on the affected side[9].

Phlebography with the limb in relaxed position and in the inciting positions will confirm the obstruction to flow.

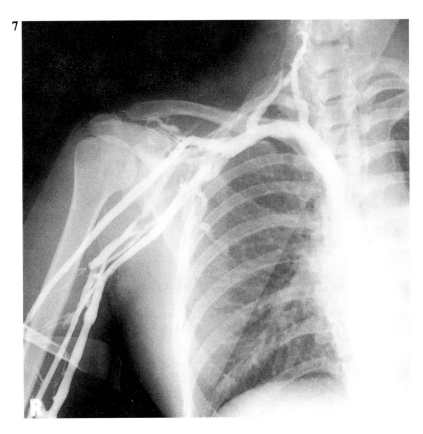

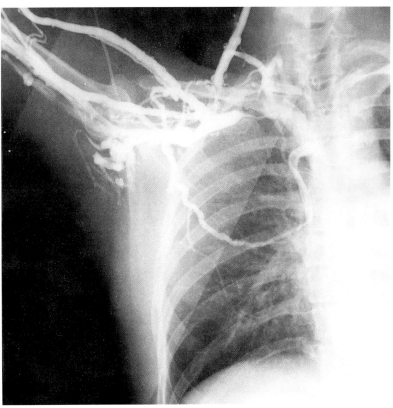

7 This young woman complained of intermittent tiredness and fullness in the arm during any exercise which involved elevating the arms. The vein was unobstructed when the arm was at the side.

8 Abduction of the arm resulted in obliteration of flow where the vein crossed the first rib. Previous supraclavicular exploration and scalenotomy had failed to relieve the symptoms.

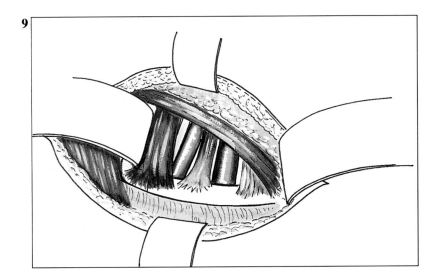

9 The anatomical relations of the subclavian artery and vein as they cross the first rib. This is the conformation seen in the axillary aproach to first rib resection. The patient is lying on the left side with the right arm abducted to approximately 90 degrees.

Towards the left of the picture the scalenus medius muscle inserts into the upper surface of the posterior part of the shaft of the first rib. Anterior to that can be seen the T1 root of the branchial plexus and the subclavian artery. Scalenus anterior separates the artery from the subclavian vein. To the right of the vein can be seen the costoclavicular ligament.

The 'scissors', the blades of which are formed by the clavicle and the first rib, have been opened by the elevation of the arm. The upper blade, the clavicle, arches across the top of the field obscured by fat and the subclavius muscle. Deep to these structures is the apex of the lung and the suprapleural membrane which is attached to the inner border of the rib. An excellent description of the operation of first rib resection has been provided by Roos[11].

First rib resection

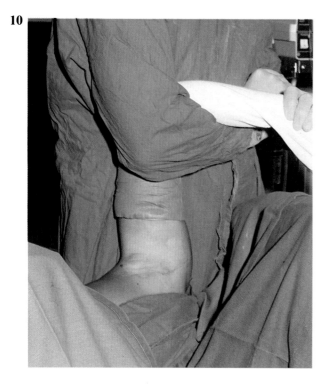

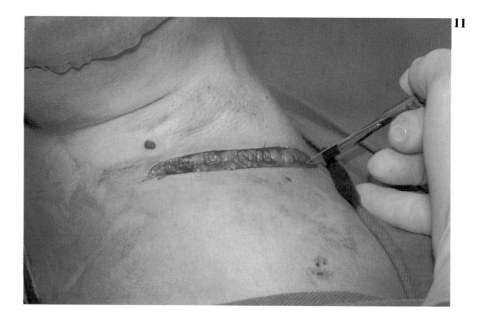

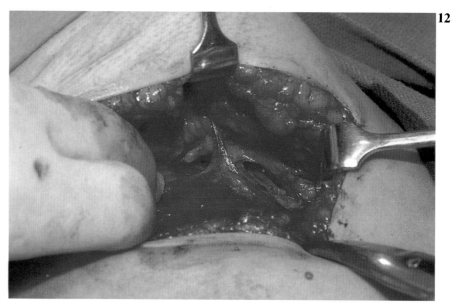

10 The patient's arm is held by the second assistant in a double wrist lock. This is safer and more effective than mechanical fixation of the arm. The assistant opens up the axilla by elevation of the limb when the surgeon is working, relaxing at intervals to ensure that there is no prolonged stretching of the brachial plexus.

This patient has undergone a previous scalenectomy which had failed to relieve outlet compression symptoms.

11 The skin incision of approximately 10 cm in length is made transversely over the third rib, below the hairline.

12 It is extended straight down to the rib cage where an areolar tissue plane is found.

13 After ligation of the thoracoepigastric vein, the plane is developed upwards to the first rib. The intercostobrachial nerve, visible adjacent to the forceps, is preserved if possible. The supreme intercostal artery and vein are ligated. The long thoracic nerve is avoided and protected.

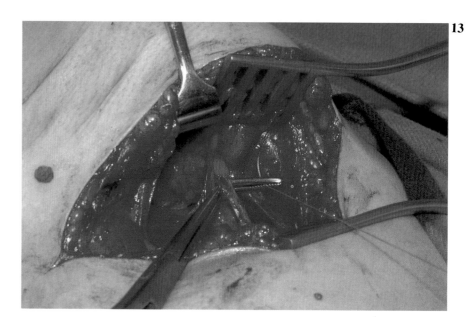

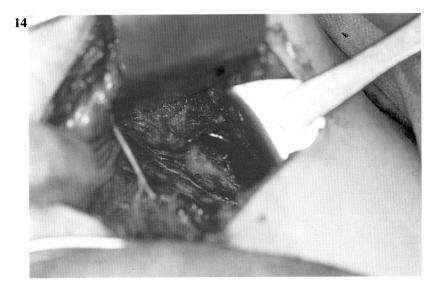

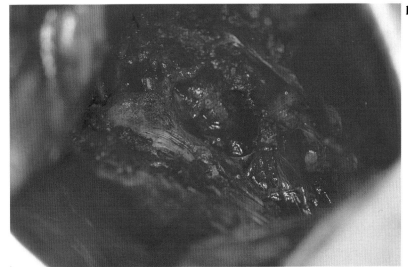

14 The upper border of the first rib is defined by blunt dissection and the sublavian vessels and branchial plexus separated off gently. Elevation of the shoulder by the second assisstant now opens up the thoracic outlet. **Great care is taken to avoid retraction on the brachial plexus.** The main retraction is anteriorly on the pectoral muscles. In this case the anatomy was difficult to define (and to photograph) because of the previous surgery. The medial part of the upper border of the first rib has been freed. Despite the previous scalenotomy there is muscle and tendon still attached to the scalene tubercle. To the left of the tubercle the subclavian artery is passing upwards and to the left disappearing under the blade of the retractor.

The subclavius tendon is felt as a taut cord anterior to the vein. It is dissected free by spreading with long scissors in the direction of the tendon, **utmost care being taken to avoid damage to the vein. Major haemorrhage is unlikely in experienced hands but should it occur, the surgeon must be prepared to deal with it rapidly by a supraclavicular approach. Generous cross-matching and the availability of vascular instruments are wise precautions.**

15 The tendinous insertion of the scalenus anterior muscle is divided at this stage. A portion of the divided tendon can be seen. The scalenus medius muscle and the first intercostal muscles are separated from the rib. The periosteum should not be elevated but should be removed with the rib. The pleura is stripped from the under surface of the rib and it can usually be kept intact avoiding the need for chest drainage.

The suprapleural membrane and other remnants are cleared from the inner border of the rib by means of a raspatory, thus freeing the rib from the transverse process of the vertebra to the costal cartilage anteriorly.

16 The rib is divided posteriorly with rib shears. This is made easier if the blades of the shears have an angle of 90-degrees. To protect the brachial plexus the nerves are being pushed up away from the shears by means of a retractor.

17 The anterior end of the rib is now divided at the costochondral junction. The stumps are smoothed with a rongeur to avoid damage to nerves or vessels. The thoracic outlet is searched carefully for any other cause of compression.

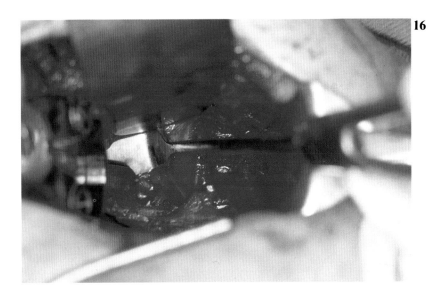

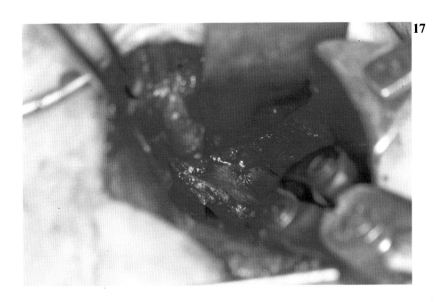

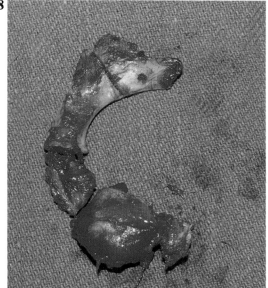

18 Excised first rib.

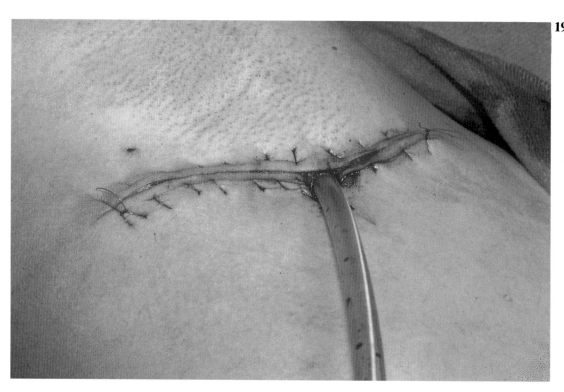

19 If the pleura appears to be intact its integrity is checked by irrigation with saline. If there is any leak, a chest drain is brought out through the rent, over the second rib and through the centre of the wound.

The chest drain may be removed in the recovery room if there is no continuing air leak and if an erect chest film shows full expansion.

Postoperative care comprises standard chest physiotherapy, pain control and gentle shoulder exercises.

13 Chronic Venous Insufficiency and the Post-thrombotic Syndrome

This group of chronic venous disorders forms a spectrum of clinical features which at one extreme are purely due to valvular insufficiency and at the other are the result of venous obstruction. If VALVULAR INCOMPETENCE is the problem, then it is the skin and subcutaneous tissues of the gaiter area which are mainly affected. The manifestations of chronic venous insufficiency include inflammation, induration, scarring (collectively known as lipodermatosclerosis), pigmentation, eczema and ulceration (see Chapter 14). These manifestations can develop as the result of incompetence in the superficial system alone[1-3] but in the majority the deep veins and perforators are also incompetent[4,5]. If OBSTRUCTION OF THE DEEP VEINS is the main lesion, then swelling, heaviness and claudication (the post-thrombotic syndrome) are the dominant symptoms.

Most patients are treated conservatively with weight reduction, skin care, elevation of the limb at rest and, most important, the encouragement of mobility combined with graduated elastic compression (page 114).

The role of surgery in chronic venous insufficiency is controversial but it has a worthwhile place in carefully selected patients. There are two broad strategies:
1 Perforator ligation.
2 Venous reconstruction.

Ligation of perforators

The varicose veins which accompany chronic venous insufficiency differ from uncomplicated primary varicose veins in a number of respects. They tend to be extensive, friable and embedded in chronic inflammatory tissue. Incompetent perforators underlie the areas of inflammation in the lower calf where the anatomy may be obscure and dissection difficult.

While the superficial veins in the thigh and upper calf can be dealt with in broadly the same way as described for primary varicose veins, a different approach may be required for the perforators. For the reasons given above, the operation is better done under tourniquet.

If the skin changes are not too advanced it may be possible, and cosmetically preferable, to deal with the perforators extrafascially through small incisions. This can either be done by direct dissection ligation (see Chapter 6, Fig. **19**), which is the author's preference, or blindly by passing a 'phlebotome' down the extrafascial plane.

But where the chronic inflammation and ulceration has produced a layer of solid, vascular scar tissue between skin and deep fascia, the choice is between non-surgical treatment or a subfascial approach to the perforators.

Subfascial ligation

Ulcers and eczema should be healed by a period of hospital in-patient treatment, if necessary, before vein surgery is attempted. Any sources of proximal incompetence are dealt with first by the techniques described earlier. The wounds are closed, the leg exsanguinated with Esmarch bandage or Rhys-Davies exsanguinator, a thigh tourniquet is applied and the patient is positioned prone.

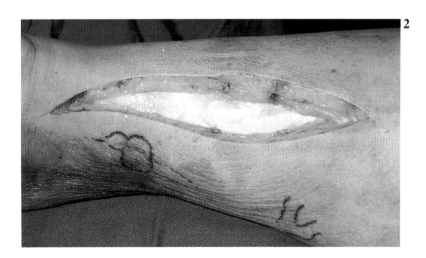

1 Where the lipodermatosclerosis is not very dense, a posteromedial incision (similar to that described by Cockett[6] for extrafascial ligation) may be satisfactory. Usually a posterior 'stocking seam' (Linton) incision is preferred[7]. This gives access to both lateral and medial perforators. It curves off the tendo achilles at its lower end to whichever side has the lowermost perforators, usually the medial side.

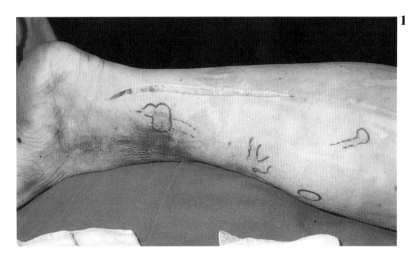

2 No attempt is made to dissect out superficial veins and care is taken not to undermine the skin flaps. The incision is carried down through the deep fascia which, in this picture, is still intact.

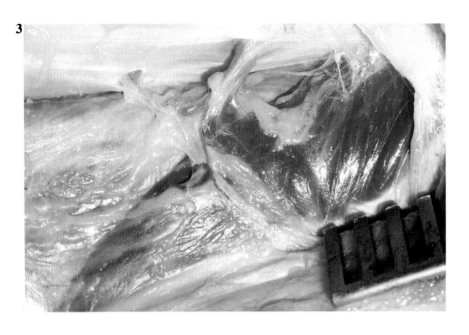

3 The muscles are separated, mainly with finger dissection, from the under surface of the fascia which is raised to reveal the perforators. This close-up view shows a large and a small perforator.

4 Ideally, to safeguard skin healing one should separate and preserve the tiny arteries which accompany the perforators. This is seldom possible in practice.

5 The perforators are ligated and divided. A careful search is made further afield for other perforators. There is often one high up the medial calf which can be ligated or clipped without unduly extending the incision.

The deep fascia is left unsutured as a fasciotomy but the skin[2] is carefully and accurately closed with a continuous monofilament or a synthetic absorbable suture without tension. The leg is bandaged before the tourniquet is released.

6 The wound at four days. Subcuticular closure gives a satisfactory cosmetic result.

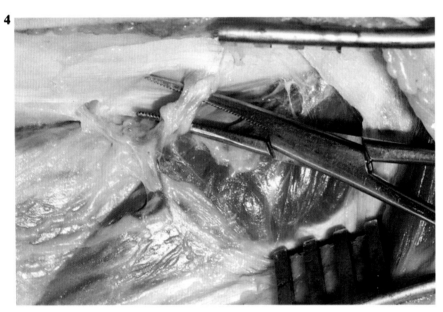

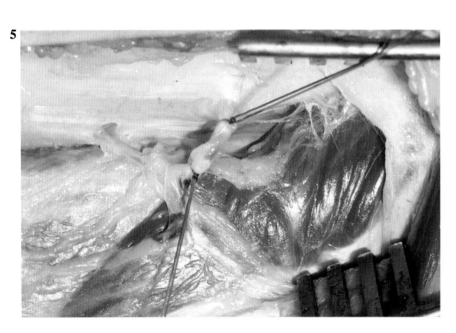

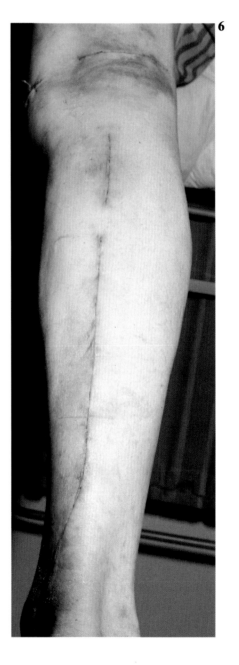

Aftercare

7 The patient is nursed with the leg elevated for several days.
Because healing is sometimes precarious, mobilisation is slow
and cautious. Low dose subcutaneous heparin, 5,000 u tid, is
started pre-operatively and continued until the patient is freely
ambulant. A lightweight knee-length graduated compression
stocking is fitted before the patient leaves hospital and may
require to be continued longterm.

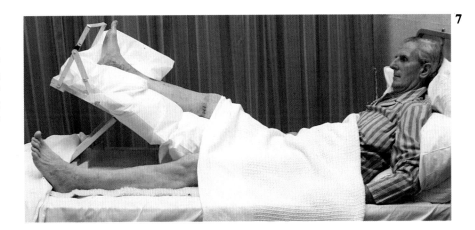

Venous reconstruction

Obstructed veins can be bypassed and incompetent valves can be
repaired[8-10] or replaced[11-13]. The latter techniques are currently
being evaluated in a few centres around the world and cannot yet be
recommended for general application. Vein bypass operations on
the other hand have a definite but limited place. They may be
considered on the rare occasions when symptoms of venous outflow
obstruction cannot be relieved by conservative measures.

Valve reconstruction

This type of surgery has been pioneered notably by Kistner[8].
Because it is only applicable to 5 per cent or less of the population of
patients with chronic venous disease, careful patient selection is
most important. It may be considered in patients who have a severe
syndrome of chronic venous insufficiency, who have been shown by
descending phlebography to have extensive deep valve
incompetence and in whom simpler measures have proven
ineffective. The operation involves a direct approach to a defective
valve through a longitudinal venotomy beginning below the valve
and repair of the cusps under direct vision. An alternative technique
via a transverse venotomy above the valve has been described by
Raju[10].

Valve transplantation

The alternative to repairing a valve is transposition of a segment of
vein containing a healthy valve. For example, if the superficial
femoral vein is incompetent but the profunda is competent, the
divided superficial femoral can be anastomosed to the profunda
below the competent valves. Good results have been reported with
this procedure[9].

Taheri has reported successful results obtained by transplanting a
2 cm segment of brachial vein containing a functioning valve into
the popliteal vein[13].

Most accounts of venous valve reconstruction report encouraging
early results. **However, vein surgery continues to carry a high
thrombosis rate, while attempts to correct this with aggressive
anticoagulant regimens incur an appreciable morbidity from bleeding
complications.** Whether these operations can be recommended for
general adoption will depend on the results after many years of
follow up. Difficult as they would be to conduct, this is an area in
which controlled clinical trials should be seriously considered.

Venous bypass

Obstructed deep veins can be bypassed using either vein or
synthetic material. Externally supported PTFE (page 36) appears to
be the synthetic material of choice at present. To avoid
re-thrombosis there must be a substantial pressure gradient to
ensure high volume flow through the graft. For this reason some
surgeons add an arteriovenous fistula which is closed 6 weeks later.

The Palma operation

The best known and most successful example of vein bypass is the Palma saphenous femoro-femoral crossover graft for iliac vein obstruction[14]. The indications are well defined and uncommon. The patient presents with a post-thrombotic swollen leg, venous claudication and bursting sensations aggravated by elastic compression. Radiologically the principal occlusion must be at iliac level. The distal pressure must be shown to rise on exercise. There must be good venous inflow up to the level of the common femoral on the affected side.

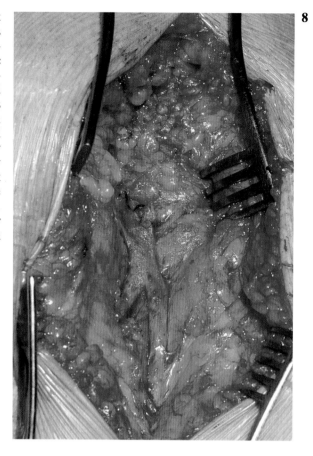

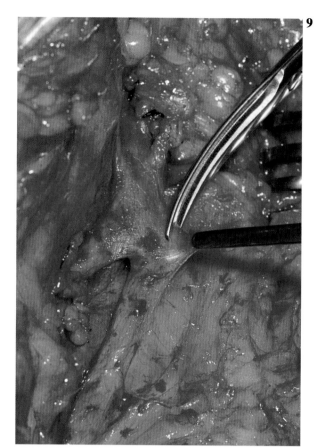

8 The saphenofemoral junction on the affected side is explored first.

9 It is cleaned of adventitia.

10 If there is doubt about the patency of the femoral vein, slings are applied and it is opened at this stage. Note the avoidance of metal jawed clamps.

11 Any webs or adhesions within the vein are excised with fine scissors.

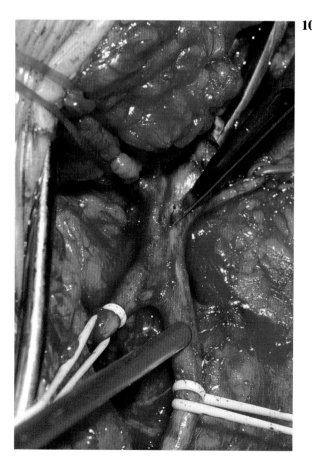

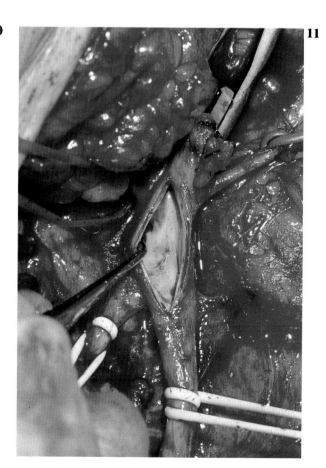

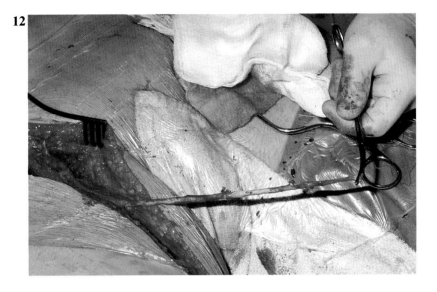

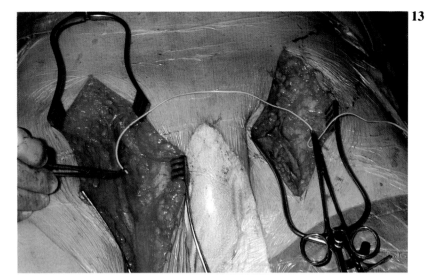

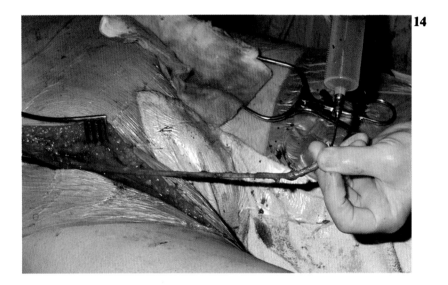

12 The contralateral long saphenous vein, which must be disease-free and of good calibre, is mobilised down to the knee. Its tributaries are flush-ligated with fine silk.

13 The length of vein required is checked.

14 The vein is gently irrigated with heparinised isotonic saline.

15 A suprapubic tunnel is made with the fingers approaching from either side.

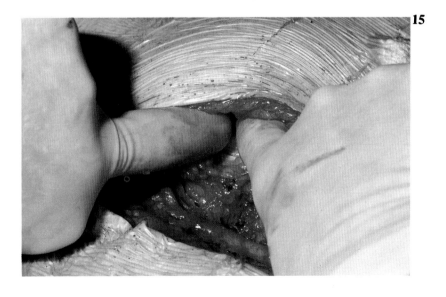

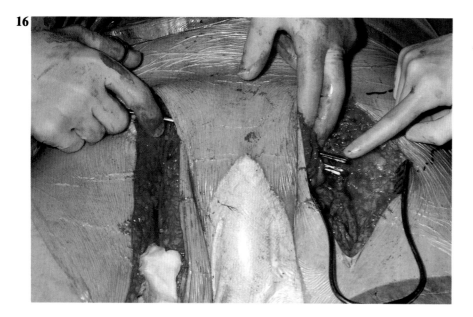

16 Mid line fascia is pierced with sponge-holding forceps.

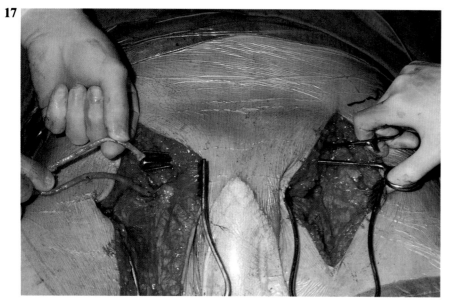

17 The saphenous vein is tunnelled subcutaneously across to the saphenofemoral junction of the affected side. During this manoeuvre great care is taken not to twist the vein.

18 The saphenous vein arches up from the saphenofemoral junction on the donor side without kinking. Note the deep external pudendal artery crossing below the junction.

19 The distal end of the long saphenous vein is shaped for anastomosis by first opening it longitudinally for 2-3 cm.

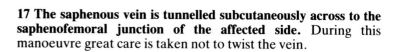

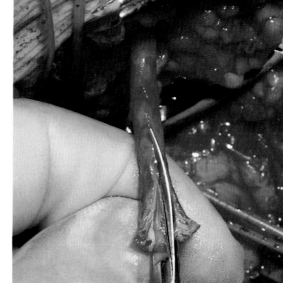

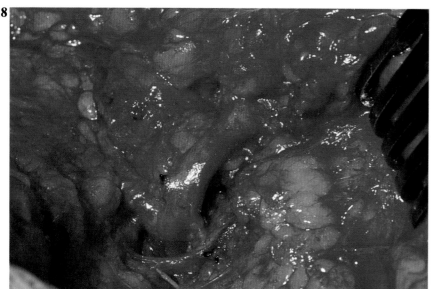

20 The corners are bevelled.

21 Using fine monofilament the transposed long saphenous is anastomosed end-to-side on to the bulb of recipient long saphenous just where it turns through the foramen ovale to join the femoral vein. Alternatively, the saphenous may be anastomosed directly to the femoral vein. **Great care must be taken to avoid undue tension or kinks.** The heel and the back row of the anastomosis is constructed with a 'purse-string' continuous monofilament suture. A nerve hook is used to hold the multiple loops of the purse-string. Note that the surgeon is holding the vein in his fingers, this being less traumatic than forceps.

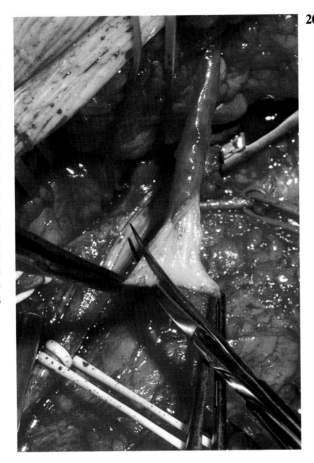

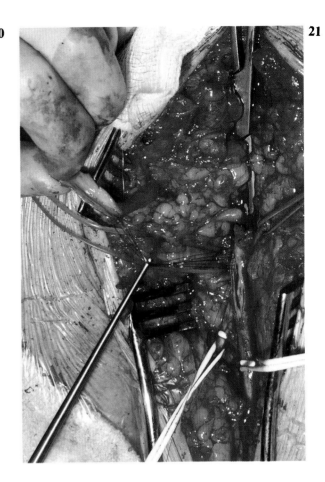

22 The purse-string is tightened down.

23 The monofilament is continued down the anterior margin of the anastomosis.

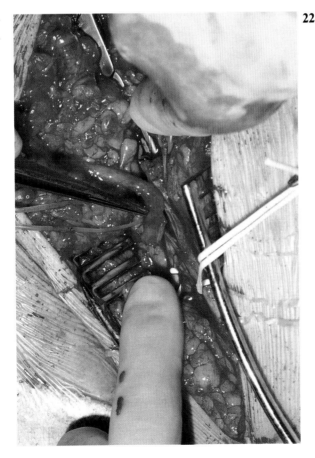

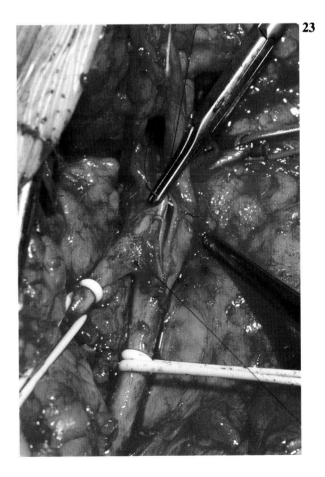

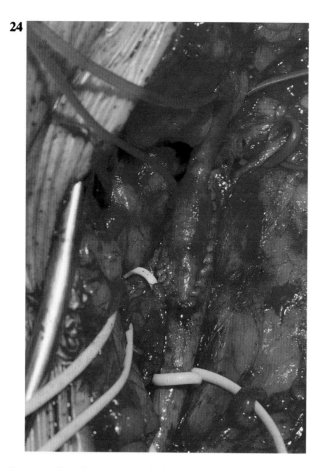

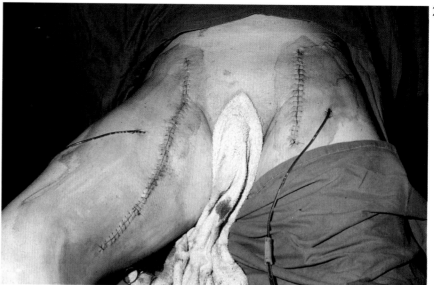

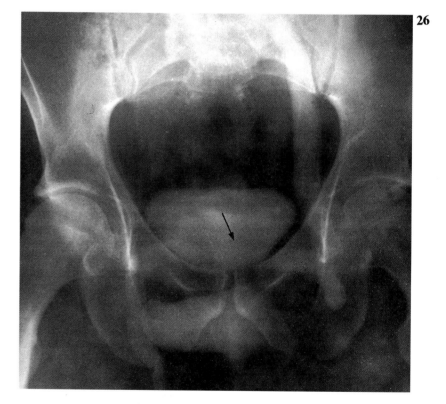

24 Here the completed anastomosis is shown. In this operation the saphenous vein was anastomosed to the common femoral vein. The anastomosis should be a long one. This appears to ensure better patency.

25 The wounds are closed over vacuum drains.

It has not usually been the author's practice to add an arteriovenous fistula, but if this is thought necessary to ensure high flow, the venovenous anastomosis is constructed side-to-side and the long saphenous vein is continued on to be anastomosed end-to-side to the adjacent femoral artery. A ligature is left around this extension, tied over a button and buried just under the skin so that the fistula can be closed at 6 weeks with minimal dissection.

The patient is maintained on continuous intravenous heparin during and after operation and converted 10 days later to oral anticoagulants which are continued for at least 3 months. Postoperatively, the patient is nursed with the foot of the bed elevated for several days and is fitted with knee-length graduated compression stockings before being mobilised.

26 Palma grafts have a good record of long-term patency. This patient had a graft constructed 14 years previously for a right iliac occlusion. The transposed left long saphenous vein is arrowed.

14 Chronic Leg Ulcers

Introduction

1 Approximately 1 per cent of the adult population suffer from chronic ulcers of the legs[1-3].

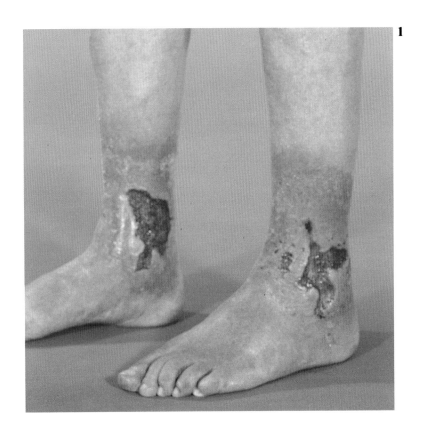

The following graphs are derived from the Lothian and Forth Valley leg-ulcer project in which 600 patients with 827 ulcerated legs were studied[4,5].

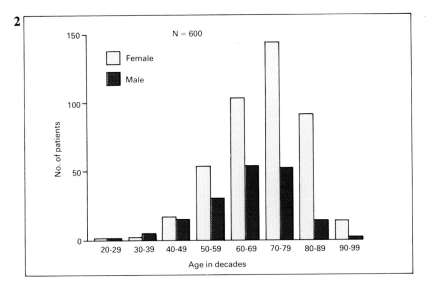

2 The condition is rare below 40 years of age; the prevalence rises sharply with age to peak in the 70-79 years of age group. Ulcers are more common in women with an overall ratio of 2.8:1 but this difference is particularly striking in the older age groups. Below 50 years of age they are as common in males as in females.

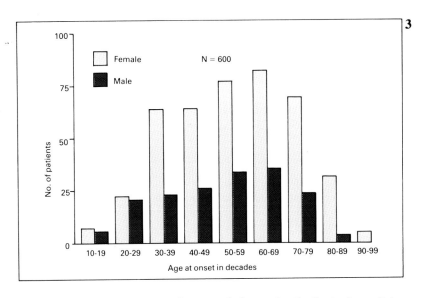

3 If one examines the age of onset of the patient's first ulcer, it is evident that this far from being a disease of the elderly.

4 Diseases associated with chronic leg ulcer are documented here for the 600 patients. Although most ulcers have several aetiological factors, some two-thirds of the patients have clinical features and/or a history of previous venous diseases of which deep vein thrombosis is the most important.

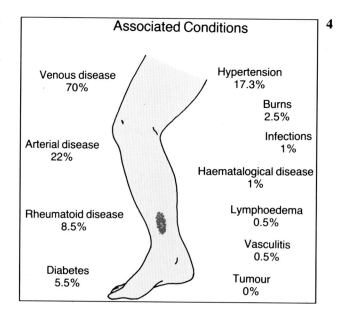

Associated Conditions

Venous disease 70%
Arterial disease 22%
Rheumatoid disease 8.5%
Diabetes 5.5%
Hypertension 17.3%
Burns 2.5%
Infections 1%
Haematalogical disease 1%
Lymphoedema 0.5%
Vasculitis 0.5%
Tumour 0%

5 These ulcers are very slow to heal. Although published series give the impression that most heal within 2 or 3 months, such series are usually based on hospital-treated patients and do not represent the whole picture. This study showed that nearly half of the ulcers took more than a year to heal. Some ulcers had remained unhealed for many years.

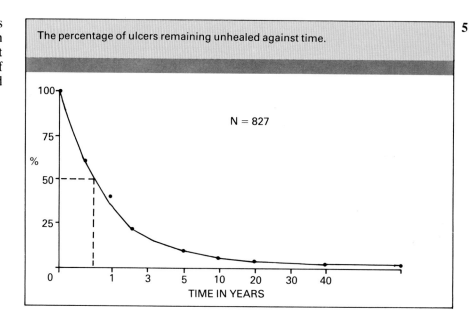

The percentage of ulcers remaining unhealed against time.

N = 827

TIME IN YEARS

6 More serious is the fact that the vast majority of ulcers recur repeatedly. This pie chart shows the number of episodes reported in relation to the 827 affected legs.

These characteristics combine to pose a very large and expensive burden on the health services. In the UK the greatest proportion of care is provided by District Nurses in the patients' homes or at Health Centres. Many physiotherapists are also skilled in the treatment of leg ulcers. While most patients can be treated on an ambulatory basis, admission to hospital may be required for more intensive treatment of the resistant or neglected ulcer. With rest, elevation and skin-grafting healing can usually be achieved. The question of surgery to the underlying venous disorder should then be considered with the aim of preventing recurrence[7-10]. The following section provides an outline of the management of the patient suffering from chronic leg ulcer.

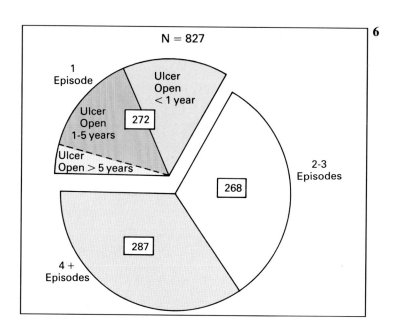

N = 827

1 Episode
Ulcer Open < 1 year
272
Ulcer Open 1-5 years
Ulcer Open > 5 years
2-3 Episodes
268
4+ Episodes
287

Diagnosis

As the cause of chronic leg ulcer is seldom single or simple, careful assessment is vital. The diagnosis of ulcer type can be made by inspection alone in some patients but in others a thorough history, examination and laboratory investigations are necessary.

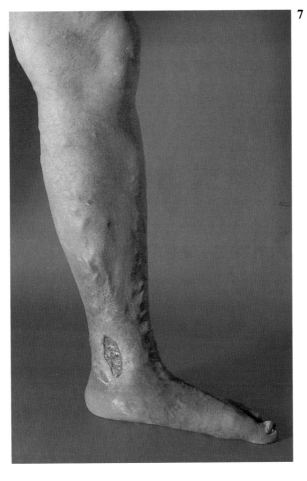

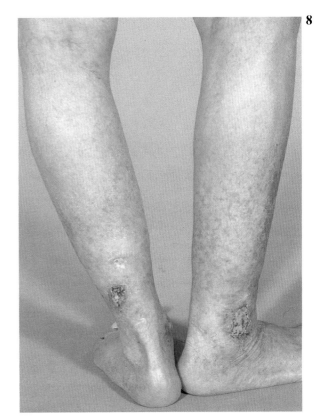

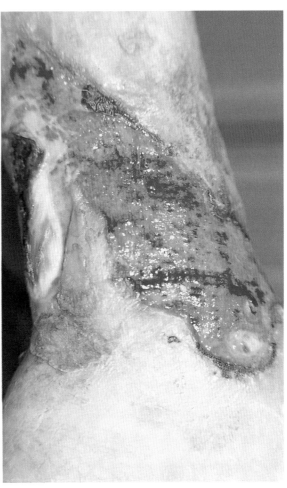

7 A venous ulcer has a number of well defined characteristics. It is typically solitary and roughly an elongated oval in shape. It lies on or posterior to the medial malleolus. Near the upper pole of the ulcer is one or more large incompetent perforating vein linking the posterior arch tributary of the long saphenous vein to the posterior tibial system. Varicose veins are usually visible in the upper calf and thigh. The surrounding skin and subcutaneous tissues show the signs of lipodermatosclerosis. If an ulcer does not conform to these features, the possibility of an unusual aetiology should be considered.

In terms of laboratory assessment chronic ulcers of venous origin are associated with ambulatory venous pressures of greater than 40 mmHg and on foot volumetry with low expelled volumes and short refilling times (Chapter 2, Fig.20).

8 The laterally placed ulcer has a different aetiology (these, for example, were arteritic). However, if venous it is likely to be associated with incompetence of lateral calf perforators and/or of the short saphenous vein.

The most important condition to exclude is ARTERIAL DISEASE. This may take two forms: atherosclerotic occlusion of large vessels or arteritis of small vessels. **It is important to detect arterial insufficiency so as to avoid inappropriate and potentially dangerous treatment such as compression bandaging**[6]. Obliterative arterial disease can play a part in promoting ulceration at any site, but it should be particularly suspected if the lesion extends on to the foot or involves pressure areas.

9 Note here the absence of lipodermatosclerosis around this arterial ulcer and its depth with exposure of the tendo achilles. The ulcer was converted from a minor skin lesion to its present serious state by application of an elastic bandage.

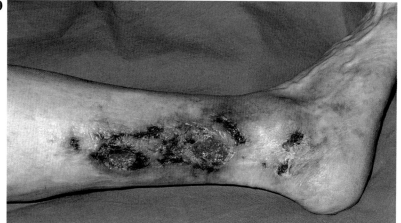

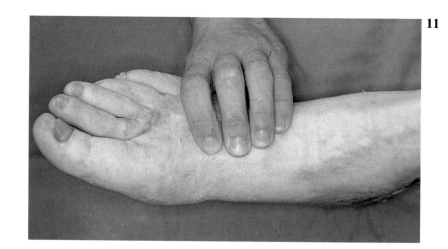

10 This ulcer began with an area of infarction.

11 Palpating for the dorsalis pedis pulse. If strong pedal pulses are felt, this excludes significant arterial disease. The posterior tibial pulse may be obscured by oedema or inflammation.

12 and 13 If the pulse is not easily felt, then the pedal pressures should be measured with Doppler ultrasound at the sites shown.

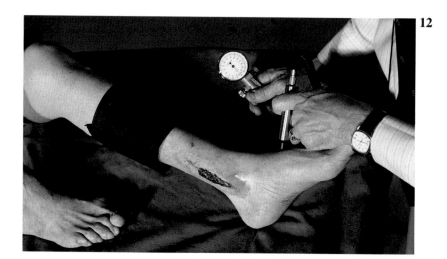

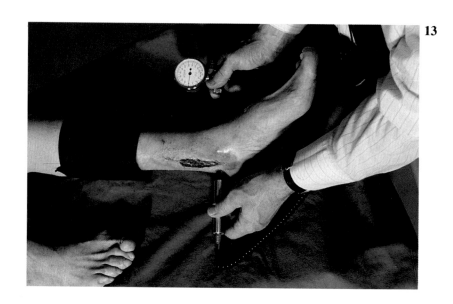

Arterial ulcers tend to be deep and more prone to cellulitis than other varieties of ulcer, especially if DIABETES is present, in which case neuropathy may also play a part.

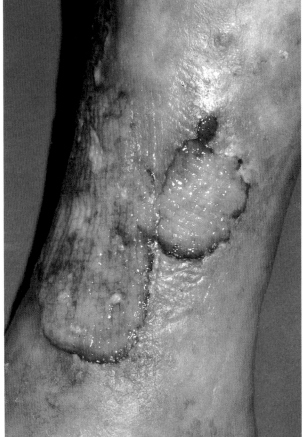

14 Arteritic ulcers are typically multiple, irregular and painful. They are frequently located on the anterior or lateral aspects of the mid or lower calf. The surrounding skin is thin and atrophic and free of lipodermatosclerosis. The clinical features of systemic autoimmune disease may be present.

15 The commonest associated disease in this group is rheumatoid. Appropriate serological tests should be part of the initial assessment of patients with atypical leg ulcers.

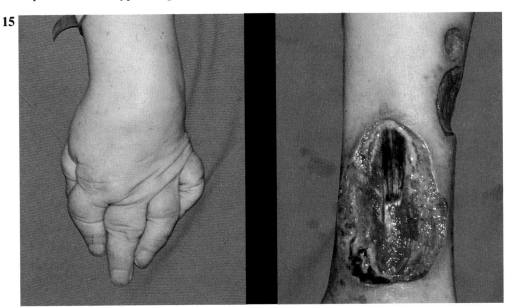

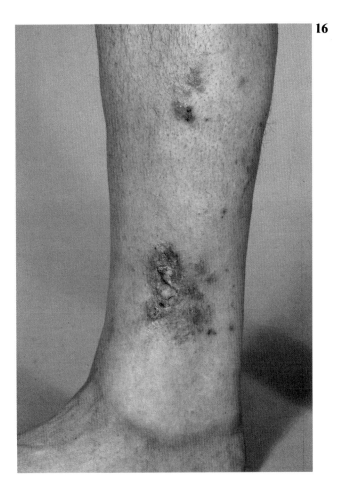

16 Chronic lymphoedema is not usually associated with ulceration unless venous insufficiency or sepsis is also present. This lesion began with an episode of streptococcal cellulitis.

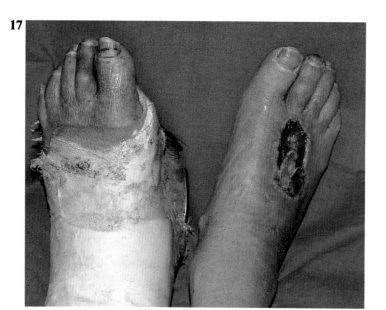

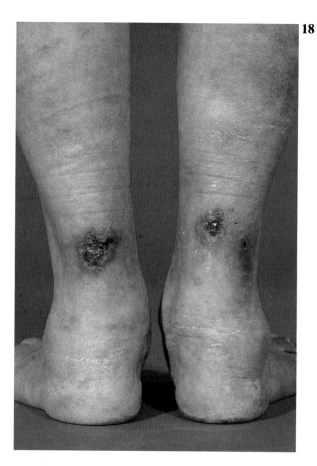

17 Most ulcers begin with minor trauma. For some the aetiology is predominantly TRAUMATIC or FACTITIAL and these are usually pretibial or on the dorsum of the foot. The patient's plaster cast rocker caused the lesion on the right foot as he slept, well sedated with alcohol. The ulcer subsequently became chronic through neglect.

18 This patient with rheumatoid disease wore high boots which chafed the back of both calves.

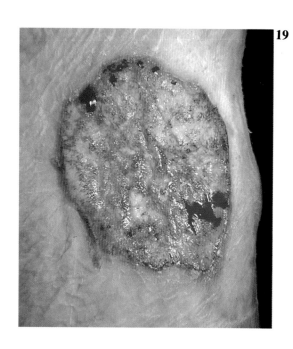

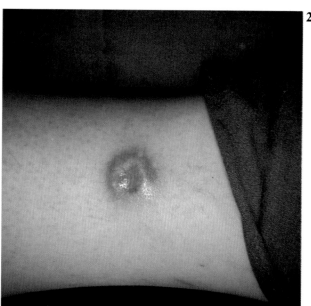

19 Malignant change in an ulcer is extremely rare. It should be suspected if chronic ulceration supervenes on scarring as a result of trauma or burn. Squamous carcinoma should also be considered if the lesion shows a poor response to conservative measures or grafting and a greater readiness to bleed than benign ulcer. The nodule silhouetted on the right alongside this ulcer was a secondary deposit.

20 This melanoma which had ulcerated shows a heaped-up edge which is typical of skin malignancy.

Care of the whole patient

Many patients with chronic leg ulcer have associated problems which play an important causative role and which may make it difficult to achieve healing. They can be divided into systemic diseases and disorders of locomotion. Among the systemic conditions are obesity, anaemia, diabetes, hypertension and autoimmune disorders. Defects of locomotion include arthropathies and neuromuscular disorders.

Thus, a general assessment of the patient is essential so that concurrent disorders may be treated. Patients with chronic leg ulcers not uncommonly live in poor social circumstances making heating, hygiene and good nutrition difficult to maintain.

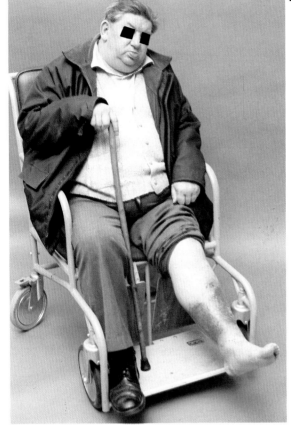

21 The control of obesity can make a crucial contribution to ulcer healing. If patients can be persuaded to lose weight and to discard corsets and girdles, a potent aggravation of venous hypertension is removed.

Care of the limb

22 Disorders of joints are common in this group of patients. The patient with chronic ulcer tends to adopt a poor gait with reduced ankle mobility and loss of calf muscle action. Contracture of the soleus and gastrocnemius may occur because of pain, disuse and fibrosis. Many patients come to rely on a walking stick, which further inhibits proper use of the muscles and joints of the legs. The efficient function of the calf muscle pump requires a free range of movement at the ankle and to a lesser extent at the knee.

23 Deformity such as this illustrates that there are limits to what physiotherapy can achieve, especially in the elderly. However, there is no doubt that education emphasising the importance of exercise, joint mobility and elevation of the legs at rest is valuable for the majority.

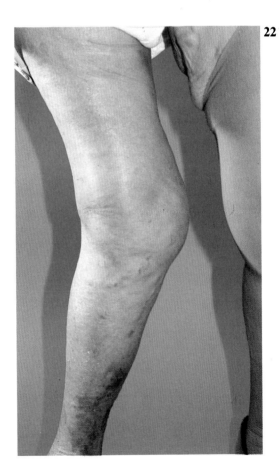

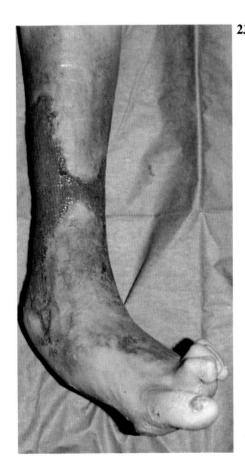

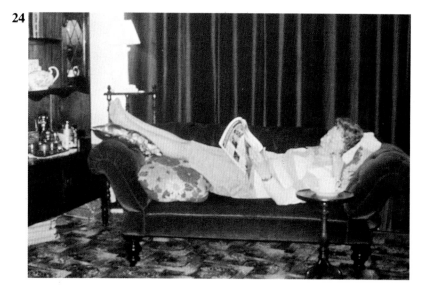

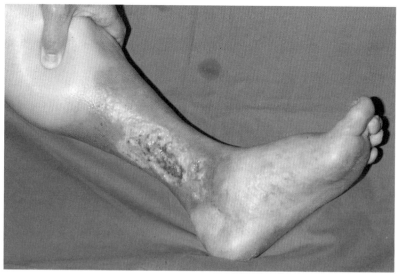

24 Of the physical measures, high elevation of the legs at rest is perhaps the most beneficial. Many elderly patients sit with their feet dependant for long periods. When elevation is recommended one often finds that this is interpreted as raising the foot for a few inches on a foot stool. **It should be made clear that elevation of the leg means that the foot must be higher than the hip.** The patient must be able to relax in comfort. At night the foot of the bed should be elevated.

25 Oedema makes ulceration almost impossible to manage because of the constant exudation. In addition to fostering bacterial proliferation the exudate causes maceration of the skin, particularly at the lower border of the ulcer. **Diuretics should not be used unless there is a specific indication such as congestive cardiac failure.** Oedema should be controlled by the simple measures outlined above. **Attempts to reduce oedema with tight bandaging are dangerous.**

Care of the ulcer

The majority of patients can remain ambulant while their ulcers are being treated. Indeed, continued use of the calf muscle pump is an important part of treatment. Only when there is frank cellulitis, severe eczema or deterioration on ambulant treatment need bed rest be considered. In this event high elevation of the leg is the crucial measure—always assuming that arterial disease has been excluded.

Whether outpatient or inpatient the nature of the ulcer dressing is of secondary importance and will be of no avail, if the underlying haemodynamic disorder is not corrected.

Caution: The healing wound needs moisture, oxygen, warmth and free drainage. All chronic ulcers are colonised with bacteria. Indeed the creation of a favourable environment for ulcer healing may also favour bacterial growth. Vigorous efforts to eradicate organisms are likely to do more harm than good.

It is vital to avoid agents which may aggravate an already unstable skin disorder. Contact dematitis, once established, is one of the most troublesome complications of chronic ulcer. Thus local antibiotics are contraindicated.

26 Here the contact dermatitis was confined to the area of the antibiotic impregnated tulle.

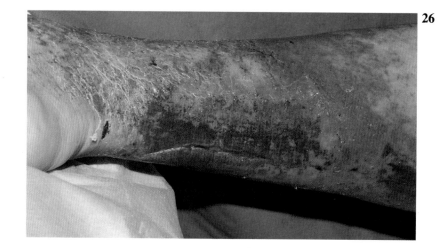

27 This allergic reaction to antibiotic spray has become generalised.

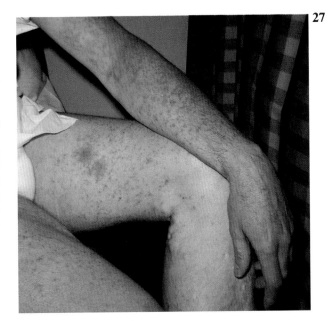

28 Paste bandage caused this reaction. Patients with possible allergies should be skin tested. It is vital that this should be expertly done in a specialist unit, because misleading results can be obtained and new sensitivities can be induced by incorrect tests. The test materials are commercially prepared in appropriate concentrations on discs.

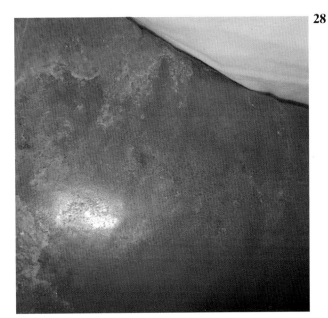

29 The discs are applied to the patient's back.

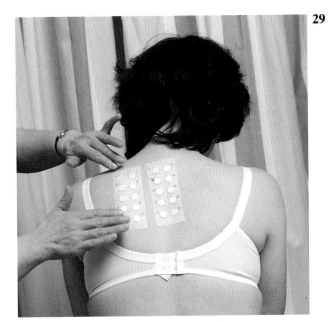

30 At 48 hours the discs are removed, the skin inspected and the position of each disc marked and labelled.

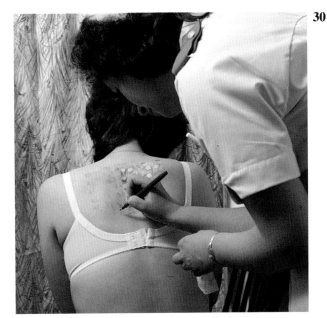

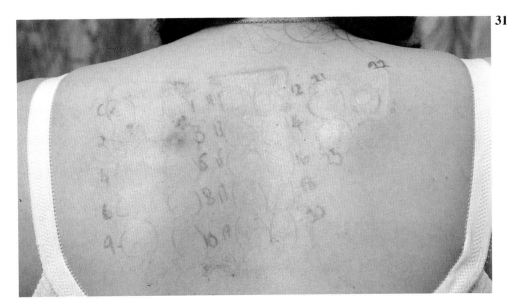

31 The sites are examined again at 96 hours. This patient has a positive reaction to one of the discs.

It is easier to say what agents should not be applied to ulcers than to make firm recommendations. The epithelial cells which grow from the edge of a healing ulcer and new granulations in the base are delicate, fragile tissues. Apart from allergic reactions, damage is also commonly done to ulcers by the application of caustic antiseptic solutions such as Eusol and Milton[11]. If used at all, these agents should be confined to the first few days of cleaning a neglected ulcer. Chemical or enzymatic desloughing agents may have their uses, although it is not proven that their efficacy justifies the cost. Partial thickness porcine dermis is an effective debriding and pain-relieving dressing which has been shown to accelerate healing[12].

Once the sloughs and crusts have been removed, a bland dressing should be preferred such as plain gauze, a synthetic non-adherent dressing, a paste-impregnated bandage, tulle gras (not antibiotic impregnated), or one of the newer hydrophilic dressings. On present evidence the choice is not critical because very few controlled trials have been reported and, as indicated earlier, healing depends mainly on the correction of the underlying haemodynamic disorder. Therefore, cost considerations become important.

Caution: Steroids should not be applied to ulcers. They do not help healing and tend to encourage colonisation by bacteria and yeasts.

The following illustrations show a system of ulcer treatment which has proven satisfactory for an outpatient clinic. The strict adherence to sterile dressing techniques is not necessary.

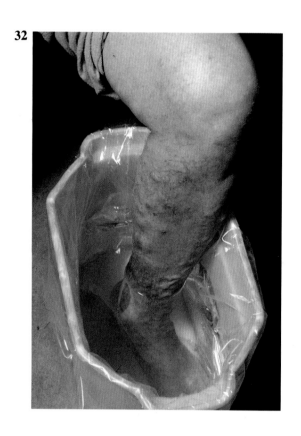

32

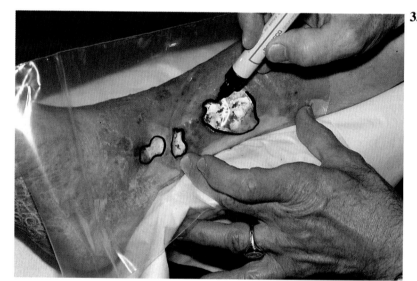

33

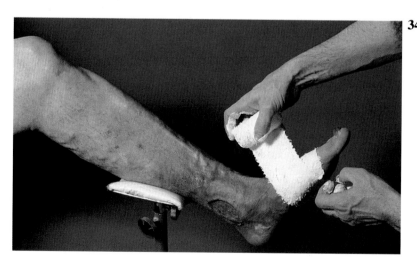

34

32 On removal of the dressing, immersion of the leg for a few minutes in lukewarm tap water is comforting and helps the removal of debris from the ulcer and surrounding skin. If there is fungal colonisation, a few crystals of potassium permanganate added to the water is a time-honoured remedy. Slough can be removed from the ulcer by gentle cleansing with water or isotonic saline on a gauze swab.

33 The area of the ulcer is traced on to transparent film so that the progress of healing can be monitored on successive visits.

34 Probably the best all-round dressing for chronic leg ulcers is the paste-impregnated bandage. It achieves its effect not only by its ingredients but by providing sustained counterpressure against oedema and by preventing slippage of the overlying layers of bandage. The paste bandage begins at the base of the toes.

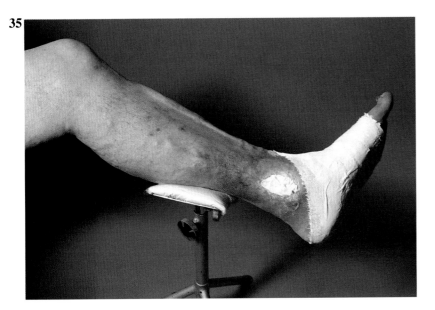

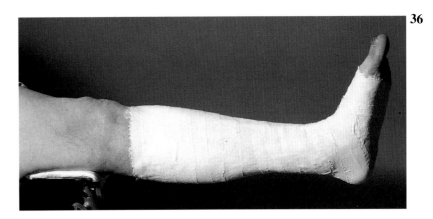

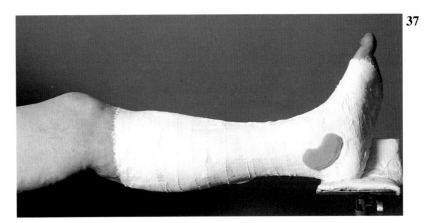

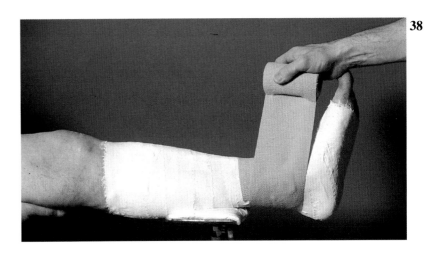

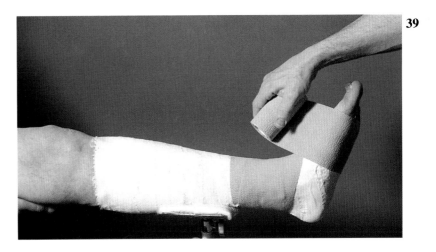

35 If an ulcer is deep, portions of bandage can be laid into it.

36 The bandage is continued up to the lower border of the tibial tuberosity.

37 For an ulcer situated in the hollow behind the malleolus, extra local pressure is brought to bear by means of a shaped piece of foam sponge.

For the patient whose skin does not tolerate paste bandages, one of the alternative dressings listed above is applied. A layer of soft absorbant bandage is added, if there is much exudate. The overlying compression bandage is applied in the same way for all dressings. The technique is shown in the following illustrations.

38 A good quality elastic bandage is applied over the paste bandage. It begins with a turn around the gaiter area.

39 It is then carried down to the base of the toes.

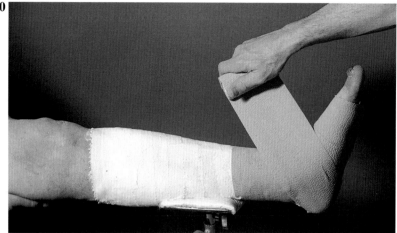

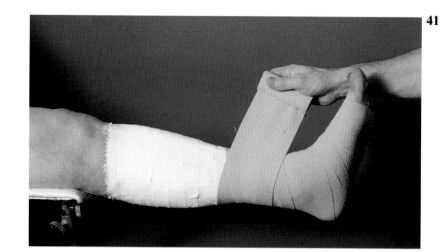

40 It is important to avoid wrinkles, especially in the ankle region.

41 Above the ankle the bandage is applied in a 'crisscross' or figure-of-eight manner with even tension.

42 The tension on the bandage is gradually reduced as it ascends the calf.

43 It is very important that those who care for leg ulcers should be skilled in bandaging techniques. For the average patient with venous ulcer, the pressure should be of the order of 30-40 mmHg at the ankle.

For most patients, but especially the heavily built individual, it pays to add a third layer of bandage, preferably of the self-adhesive variety, or a knee-length graduated compression stocking. This carries several benefits. First, it provides an extra layer for absorption of exudate. Second, it increases the compression. Third, it ensures that the underlying bandage remains securely in place. Fourth, it ensures that the compression is sustained. Compression is discussed in Chapter 16.

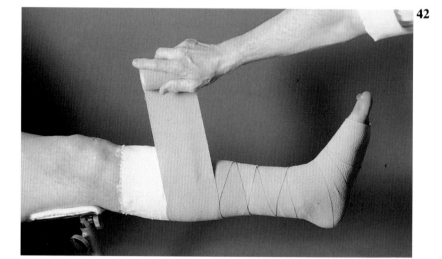

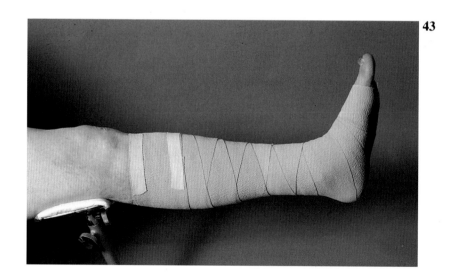

42

The FREQUENCY OF DRESSING CHANGE is determined by the amount of moist discharge. When an ulcer is in its early exudative phase, especially if the leg is oedematous, the dressings may have to be changed twice per week or even more often. It follows that the most effective way of reducing the need for frequent dressings is to control oedema by the simple physical measures outlined previously. When the exudate has started to diminish, a weekly dressing is usually sufficient.

Some patients benefit from having their treatments carried out in the physiotherapy department. Instruction in gait, exercises to improve joint mobility and muscle function, connective tissue massage to stimulate peripheral blood flow and intermittent pneumatic compression to reduce oedema may all be useful. The application of pulsed ultrasound to the indurated tissue around the ulcer accelerates healing[13].

Occasionally, surgical or chemical sympathectomy may be beneficial. It should be considered especially in those patients who have evidence of active autonomic function in the extremities as shown, for example, by sweating.

Care of the surrounding skin

44 Varicose eczema often precedes or accompanies ulcer. In its severe form it may necessitate bed-rest with elevation of the limb. Compresses of 1:10,000 potassium permanganate can be used or the leg can be painted with 2 per cent aqueous eosin. As the eczema settles, the patient is mobilised with 1 per cent aqueous hydrocortisone applied to the skin twice daily and the leg bandaged with tubegauze and a firm supporting bandage.

Contact dermatitis (pages 102) requires the removal of the sensitising agent. Patch tests are done, if there is doubt as to the cause. A 1 per cent hydrocortisone cream is usually an effective treatment.

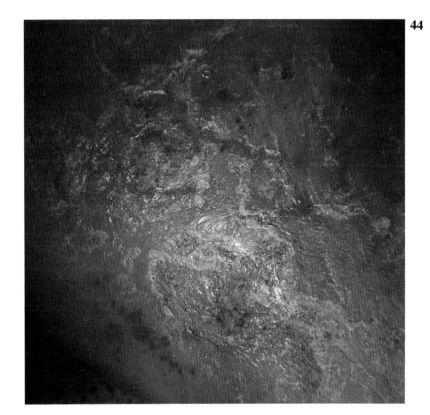

44

45 The inflammatory form of lipodermatosclerosis is often mistaken for cellulitis or phlebitis. Elevation at rest, graduated elastic compression and a course of oral Stanozolol[14] will usually control this condition and pre-empt ulceration.

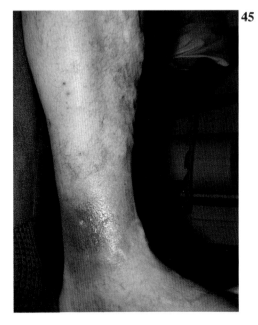

45

46 Superficial phlebitis follows the course of a varicose vein and the thrombus may be palpable. This patient had superficial phlebitis in the thigh. If mild, it should respond to elastic compression and analgesia. If severe and especially if it extends up the long saphenous vein to the groin, the likelihood of co-existing deep vein thrombosis should be considered. In such instances the patient must be referred to hospital for further investigation and heparin therapy.

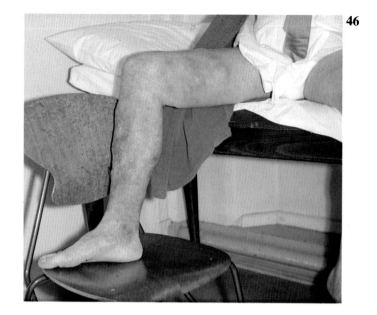

46

47 Systemic antibiotics are only indicated if there is a true cellulitis. In this case the patient will generally show systemic signs of infection.

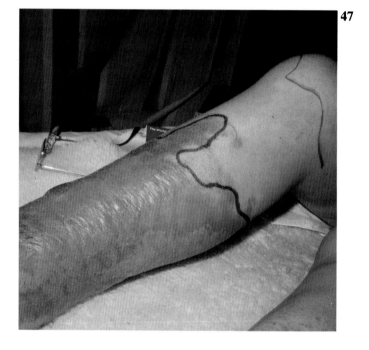

Aftercare

Virtually all ulcers can be healed by one means or another. The greater challenge is to prevent recurrence. Therefore, the patient should remain under medical supervision.

Associated disorders such as obesity should be controlled as far as possible. Patients should be encouraged to continue the physical measures of mobility combined with graduated compression (see Chapter 16) and elevation of the limb at rest. The relatively fit and mobile patient should be assessed for surgery to the underlying veins.

15   Skin Grafts

The healing of a chronic leg ulcer can be greatly accelerated by skin grafting. Although small grafts such as pinch grafts can be done on outpatients, greater success is likely to be attained with inpatient care. Before grafting is carried out a period of bed-rest is usually required, with elevation of the limb and daily dressings, to minimise exudation and bacterial colonisation and to promote healthy granulation tissue. If there is heavy bacterial colonisation, especially by haemolytic streptococcus, *Staphylococcus aureus* or *Pseudomonas pyocyaneus*, further dressings and, if necessary, systemic antibiotics should be given until a more favourable environment for grafting is obtained.

Pinch grafts

Pinch grafts have much to commend them in the treatment of chronic ulcers. Being of full thickness in the centre of each pinch they result in robust epithelial cover, able to withstand later traumas in a vulnerable area. If only a proportion of the pinches 'take', they can still make a big contribution towards healing and the gaps can be filled at a later date by further pinches, taken if necessary under local anaesthetic.

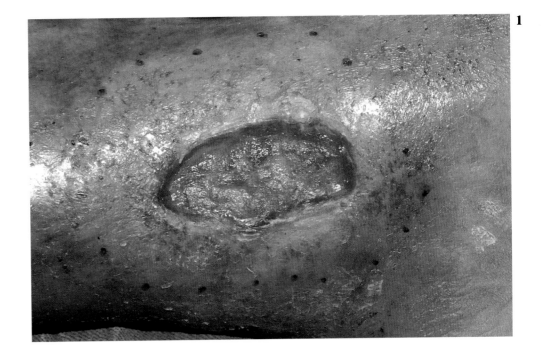

1 When this patient presented there was oedema of the limb, cellulitis, skin maceration and generalised moist eczema. The ulcer was exuding, sloughy and heavily colonised by bacteria. Outpatient treatment with paste bandages and graduated compression over 2 months brought the ulcer to the state shown.

The original dimensions of the ulcer are shown by the dotted line.

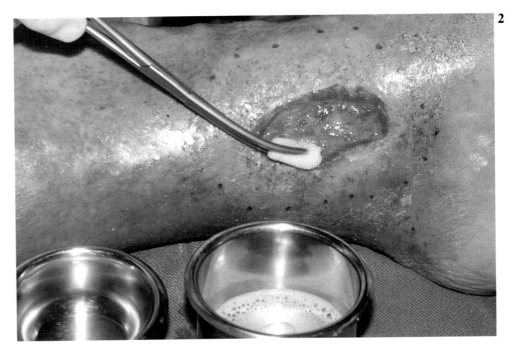

2 In theatre the ulcer surface is cleaned with cetrimide and then with isotonic saline.

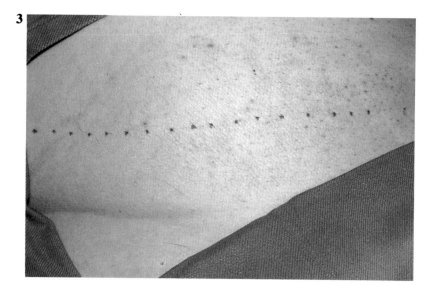

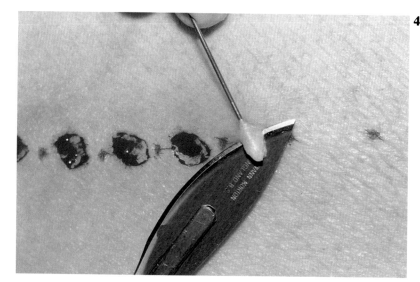

3 An area of the abdominal wall, in this case in the left iliac fossa, is prepared and a skin crease marked.

4 Pinch grafts of approximately 5 mm diameter are cut.

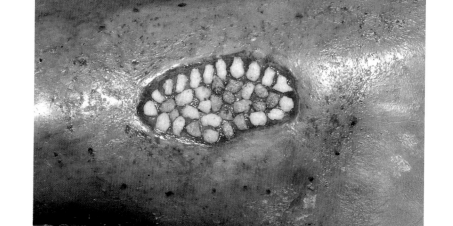

5 This ulcer has been quite well covered, but ideally the pieces of skin should be placed closer together to accelerate healing and minimise the spaces where crusting can occur.

6 A piece of tulle gras is laid over the grafted area.

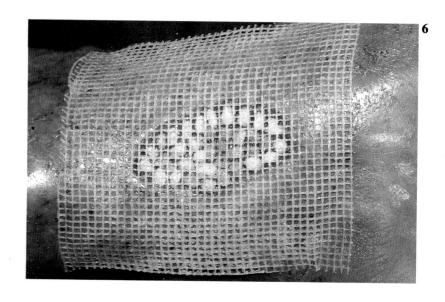

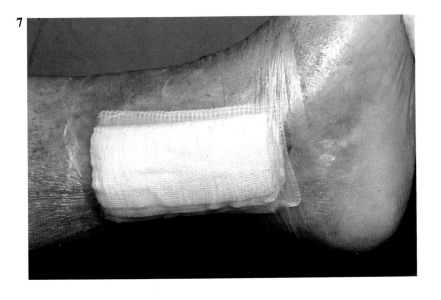

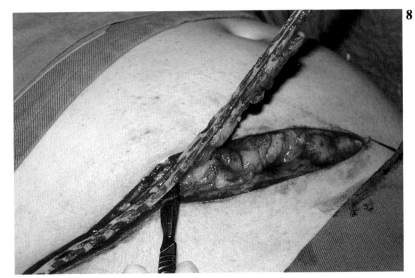

7 This is followed by a layer of gauze held in position by an adhesive dressing.

8 The donor area is excised.

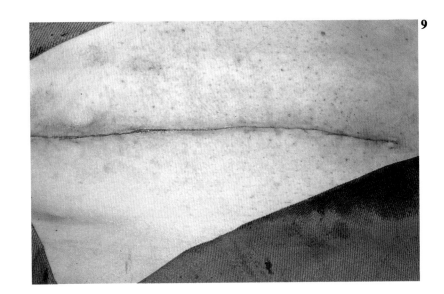

9 It is then closed with a synthetic absorbable subcuticular suture.

10 This patient had a similar graft 3 years earlier. Although cosmetically less than perfect, the excellent functional result in an area overwhelmingly prone to recurrent ulceration is well shown.

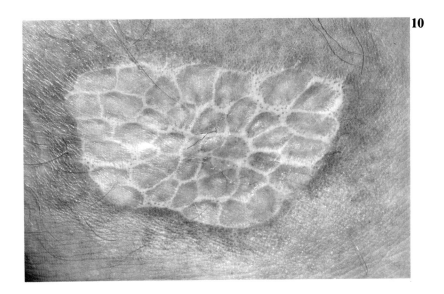

Split skin grafts

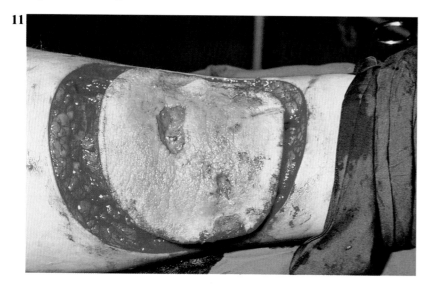

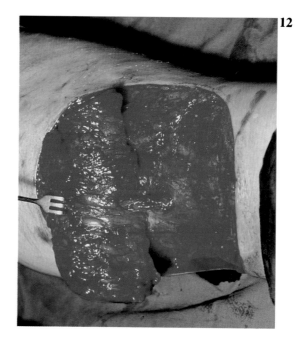

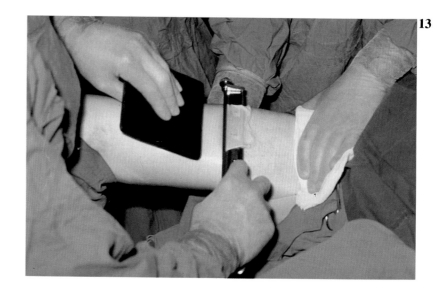

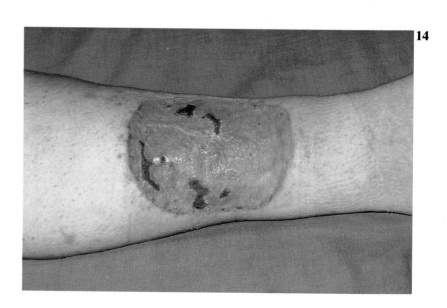

11 A large area of multiple ulcers can be excised *en bloc*.

12 The underlying surface is suitable for immediate grafting. A large perforator passes through the deep fascia in the centre of the field.

13 Split skin is taken from the thigh.

14 The appearance of the graft at 3 weeks. The small superficial defects healed without need for further grafting.

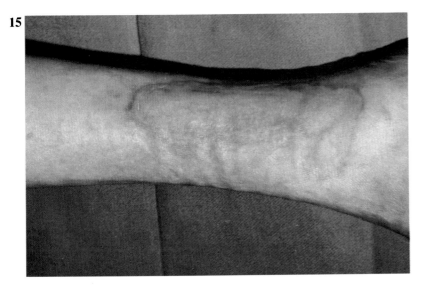

15 A similar graft at 12 months.

16 and 17   This patient had extensive bilateral ulcers grafted by this technique.

Aftercare

Skin grafting does not exempt ulcers from the almost inevitable tendency to recurrence. The comments on aftercare in the previous chapter apply equally to this group of patients.

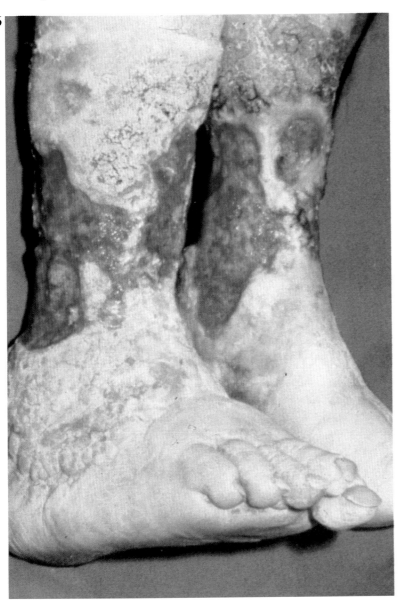

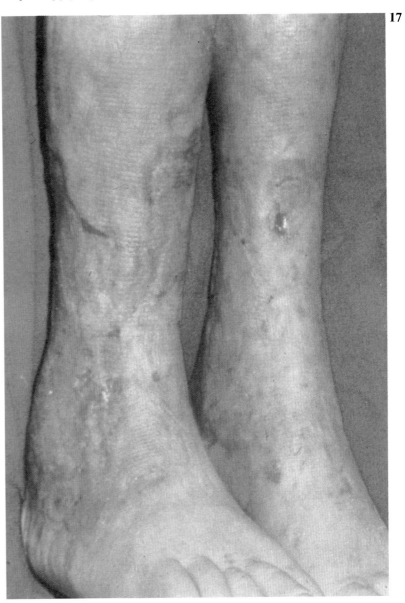

16 Compression Therapy

Compression therapy, although relegated to the last chapter, is perhaps the most important topic in the book. For every patient who is treated by operation, there are hundreds, possibly thousands, who rely on compression in various forms to ease their symptoms. In ulcer disease the compression is applied by means of bandages and in other venous disorders by means of elastic hosiery.

Compression applied to the limb, depending upon the degree of pressure, can be expected to:

1 Counteract the high pressure in superficial veins.

2 Enhance blood flow velocity in the deep veins.

3 Discourage oedema by reducing the pressure difference between the capillaries and the tissues.

The value of compression has been recognised since several centuries BC, but only very recently have scientific methods of measurement been applied to the design of compression garments and to the assessment of their physiological and therapeutic effects. A number of bench methods (for example EMPA, Hohenstein, Hatra) for measuring the tension in a material in response to a given amount of stretch have been in use by hosiery manufacturers for some time. Unfortunately, there is as yet no international agreement as to a standard reference method.

Clinicians are more interested to know what pressure the bandage or garment exerts on the leg of the individual patient and to relate this to observed benefits and to haemodynamic changes. A number of ingenious devices have been developed in recent years for direct *in vivo* pressure measurement.

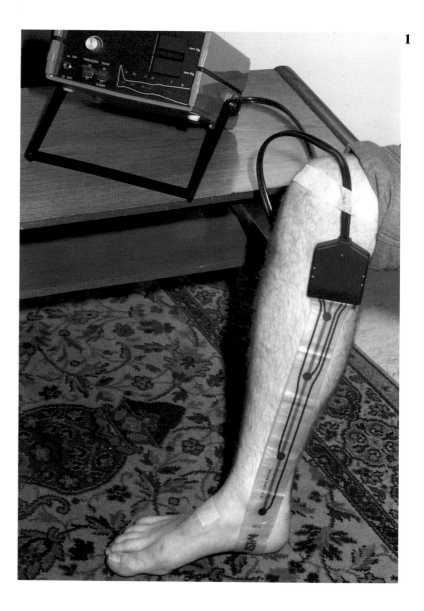

1 This Borgnis medial stocking tester is used on the patient's leg to obtain a pressure profile. The bandage or stocking is applied over the probe. The probe is connected to an electronic manometer which records the point at which inflation pressure overcomes the elastic compression. Recordings can be made at different levels up the limb.

Graduated compression

It is now recognised that the optimal haemodynamic effects are achieved when the pressure applied to a limb is in the form of a gradient which diminishes as it ascends the leg. This concept has been attributed to Conrad Jobst, an engineer, who himself suffering from venous insufficiency, in the 1950s invented a graduated compression stocking for his own use[1]. Since then, as the laboratory tools have become available, the empirical and theoretical advantages of graduated compression have been given a scientific foundation by a series of studies in the 1970s and 1980s.

For example, Sigel and co-workers (1973) used transcutaneous Doppler in the recumbent individual and demonstrated more than 100 per cent increase in blood velocity in femoral vein flow in response to graduated compression[2]. They concluded that the optimal ankle to mid-thigh pressure profile for the immobile hospital patient was 18 to 8 mmHg. The manufacturers of anti-embolism stockings have based their design on these data.

Fentem *et al.* (1976) demonstrated that well applied elastic bandages effectively emptied the superficial veins[3].

Horner *et al.* (1980) compared the effect of graduated and non-graduated compression stockings on 22 limbs with deep venous insufficiency. They found that the stockings with a graduated compression profile reduced the ambulatory venous pressure by 20 to 30 mmHg[4].

Jones and co-workers (1980) used foot volumetry and sodium isotope clearance to compare low compression (20 mmHg), medium compression (30 mmHg) and high compression (40-50 mmHg) graduated stockings and demonstrated that the physiological benefits were greatest in the high compression group[5].

The importance of these observations for the manufacture of compression stockings has been recognised. The British Standards Institution's report of 1985[6] specifies that for ankle pressures of greater than 19 mmHg the calf pressure should not exceed 70 per cent of the calf pressure as measured by the Hatra method. The pressure normally quoted by stocking manufacturers refers to the ankle level. The clinician should know precisely what he is prescribing.

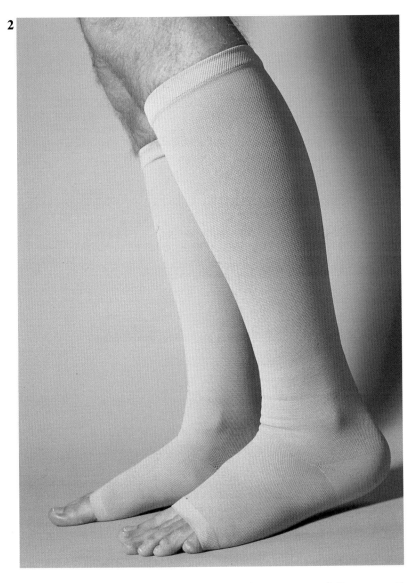

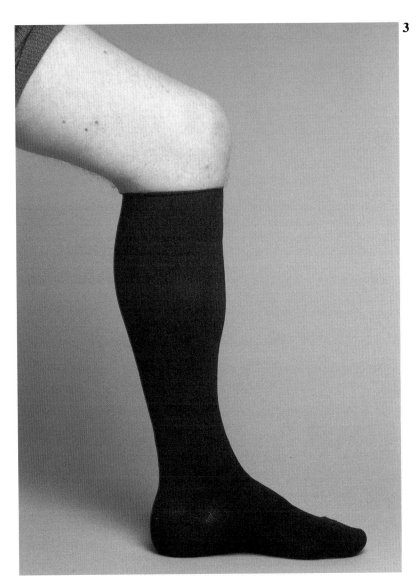

2 Full-length stockings or tights are often requested for cosmetic reasons. From a haemodynamic point of view the compression seldom needs to be applied above the knee, unless there is severe post-phlebitic syndrome or lymphoedema with swelling in the thigh. Furthermore, because they are easier to put on, compliance is likely to be better with the short stockings. Careful fitting is important. The degree of pressure that is appropriate depends on the severity of the disorder and the age, build and height of the individual. A level of 30-40 mmHg at the ankle is effective and safe for most individuals[5,7,8].

3 Cosmetic acceptability is important for patient compliance. The appearances of compression hosiery have improved in recent years. For the male patient graduated compression socks are now obtainable in a variety of colours.

Bandaging

When applying a compression bandage one is trying to achieve a graduation similar to that described for stockings. Laplace's law demonstrates that for a given tension of application, the highest pressure will be exerted to the surface of the leg with the smallest radius. This means that a bandage applied up a leg with even tension will automatically provide a gradient of pressure. However, experienced bandagers seek to exaggerate this effect by reducing the tension slightly as they ascend the limb. As with stockings, a pressure of 30-40 mmHg at the ankle is effective and well tolerated by most patients.

Bandaging technique is important and seldom formally taught to nurses or medical students. **A criss-cross or figure-of-eight type of application ensures more even and better sustained pressure than a simple spiral.** An effective bandaging technique is illustrated in Chapter 14.

The average elastic bandage loses most of its compression within an hour or two of being applied[9,10]. Self-adhesive elastic bandages maintain their pressure much more effectively, as do multilayered bandages. Elastic bandages applied over a paste bandage also sustain their pressures better[9].

Concerning the degree of stretch of compression bandages, there are two schools of thought. One favours highly elastic bandages, which exert a sustained compression that does not fall greatly when the patient changes from the standing to the lying position. The other favours non-stretch or minimal stretch bandages, which exert firm counterpressure when the patient is erect but little or none when he or she is lying. The latter would appear to be safer, especially in patients with arterial impairment. The issue does not appear to have been tested by clinical trial.

Laplace's law also explains why bony and tendonous prominences such as the malleoli and the tendons around the ankle are so vulnerable to damage by compression bandages.

Hazards of compression

4 When elastic bandaging is applied too tightly around an ulcerated area, it results in oedema of the foot.

It is vital to exclude peripheral arterial disease before applying elastic stockings or bandages to a limb. Pressure necrosis from this cause is all too often seen in vascular practice. Furthermore, it is far commoner than is generally appreciated, partly because it is not recognised and partly because such a large proportion of the care of patients with chronic leg ulcer takes place in the community.

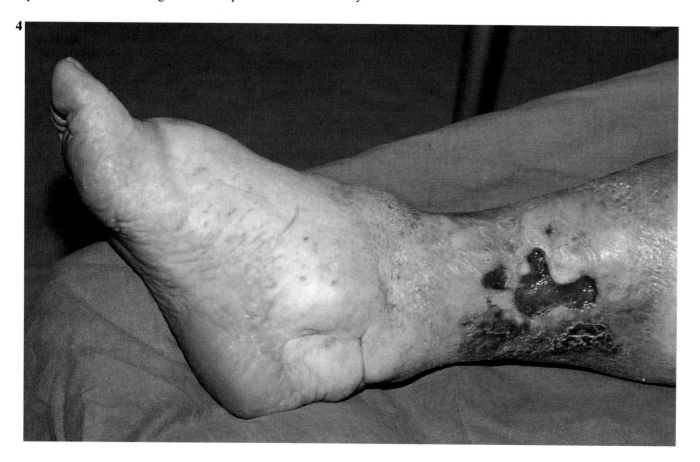

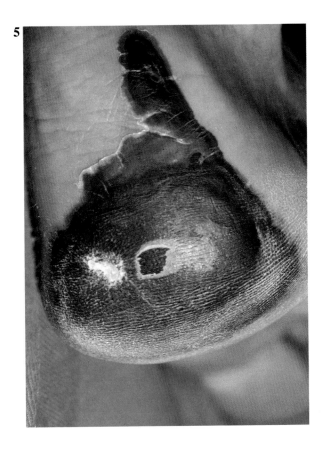

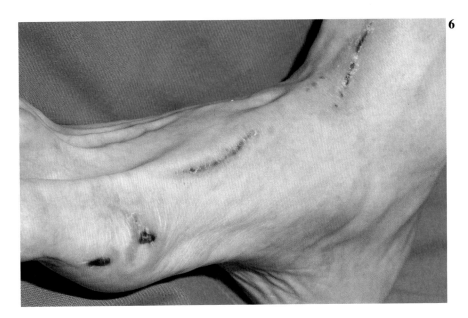

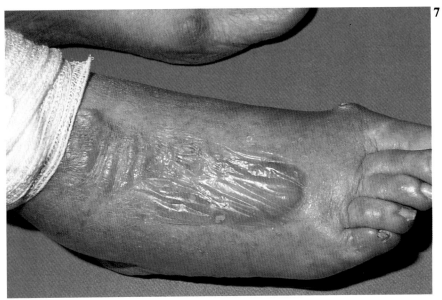

5 Elastic stockings are particularly dangerous in the patient with impaired circulation who is lying immobile in bed. The manufacturer's warnings against the application of anti-embolism stockings to patients with arterial disease were not heeded in this case.

6 Bandaging can be an even more potent cause of pressure damage. Note how, in this patient with arterial insufficiency, overtight bandaging has picked out the pressure points. A further example of bandaging damage is shown on page 116.

7 A common site for bandage-induced damage is on the front of the shin and over the tendons of the ankle.

8 This bandage-induced ulcer led to amputation.

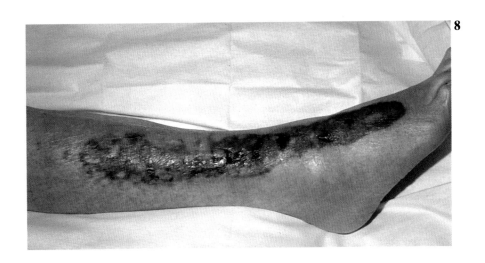

Bibliography

Chapter 1

1 Dodds H, Cockett F B. *The pathology and surgery of the veins of the lower limb*. Churchill Livingstone, London, 1976, 19-49.

2 Gardner A M N, Fox R H. The return of blood to the heart against the force of gravity. *Phlebology 85*. (Eds.) D Negus & G Jantet. Libbey, London, 1986, 65-67.

3 Lajos T Z, Espersen C. Anatomical considerations of the venous drainage of the lower extremities. *J. Surg. Research*, 1983, **34**, 1-6.

4 Lofgren P, Lofgren K A. Recurrence of varicose veins after the stripping operation. *Arch. Surg.*, 1971, **102**, 111-114.

5 Shepherd M. Incidence, diagnosis and management of sapheno-popliteal incompetence. *Phlebology 85*. (Eds) D Negus & G Jantet. Libbey, London, 1986, 94-97.

6 Mavor G E, Galloway J M G. Collaterals of the deep venous circulation of the lower limb. *S,G & O*, 1967, 561-571.

7 Sutton R, Darke S G. Stripping the long saphenous vein: peroperative retrograde saphenography in patients with and without venous ulceration. *Br. J. Surg.*, 1986, **73**, 305-307.

8 Roos D B. Surgical treatment of the thoracic outlet syndromes. In *Vascular surgery*. (Ed) C W Jamieson Baillière Tindall, 1986, 133-146.

Chapter 2

1 Rivlin S. The surgical cure of primary varicose veins. *Br. J. Surg.*, 1975, **62**, 913-917.

2 Shepherd M. Incidence, diagnosis and management of sapheno-popliteal incompetence. *Phlebology 85*. (Eds) D Negus & G Jantet. Libbey, London, 1986, 94-97.

3 Hobbs J T. Errors in the differential diagnosis of incompetence of the popiteal vein and short saphenous vein by Doppler ultrasound. *J. Cardiovasc. Surg.*, 1986, **27**, 169-173.

4 Lamont P, Bavin D, Woodyer A, Ruston M, Butler J, Terry T, Reddy P, Belli A, Dundas D, Dormandy J. Evaluation of the accuracy of clinical and Doppler examinations for detecting imcompetent perforators in patients with varicose veins. *Phlebology 85*. (Eds) D Negus & G Jantet. Libbey, London, 1986. 110-114.

5 Bjordal R I. Dilated perforated veins—a dilemma? *VASA*, 1983, **12**, 302.

6 Barnes R W. Non-invasive diagnostic techniques in peripheral vascular disease. *Am. Heart J.*, 1979, **97**, 241-258.

7 Strandness D E Jr, Sumner D S. *Hemodynamics for surgeons*, Grune & Stratton, New York, 1975.

8 Sumner D S. Physiology in venous problems. In *Surgery of the veins*. (Eds) J J Bergan & J S T Yao. Grune & Stratton, New York, 1985.

9 Thulesius O, Norgren L, Gjores J E. Foot volumetry: a new method for objective assessment of edema and venous function. *VASA*, 1973, **2**, 325-329.

10 Norgren L, Thulesius O, Gjores J E, Soderlundh S. Foot volumetry and simultaneous venous pressure measurements for evaluation of venous insufficiency. *VASA*, 1974, **3**, 140-147.

11 Lawrence D, Kakkar V V. Post-phlebitic syndrome a functional assessment. *Br. J. Surg.*, 1980, **67**, 686-689.

12 Barnes R W, Callicott P E, Sumner D S, Strandness E. Non-invasive quantitation of venous haemodynamics in the post-phlebitic syndrome. *Arch Surg.*, 1973, **107**, 807-814.

13 Pearce W H, Ricco J B, Queral L A, Flinn W R, Yao J S T. Hemodynamic assessment of venous problems. *Surgery*, 1983, **93**, 715-721.

14 Norris C S, Beyreau A, Barnes R W. Quantitative photoplethysmography in chronic venous insufficiency: A new method of non-invasive estimation of ambulatory venous pressure. *Surgery*, 1983, **94**, 758-764.

15 Albrechtsson U, Olsson C G. Thrombotic side effects of lower limb phlebography. *Lancet*, 1976, **i**, 723-724.

16 Lea Thomas M, Walters H L. Metrizamide in venography. *Br. Med. J.*, 1979, **2**, 1036.

17 Lea Thomas M, Bowles J N, Piaggio R B, Price J, Treweeke P S. Contrast agent induced thrombophlebitis following leg phlebography: Iohexol compared with meglumine iothalamate. *VASA*, 1985, **14**, 81-83.

18 Lea Thomas M. *Phlebography of the lower limb*. Churchill Livingstone, Edinburgh, 1982.

Chapter 3

1 Fegan W G. Continuous compression technique of injecting varicose veins. *Lancet*, 1963, **i**, 109-111.

2 Hobbs J T. Surgery and sclerotherapy in the treatment of varicose veins. *Arch. Surg.*, 1974, **109**, 793-796.

3 Beresford S A A, Chant A D B, Jones H O, Piachaud D, Weddell J M. Varicose veins: a comparison of surgery and injection/compression sclerotherapy. *Lancet*, 1978, **i**, 921-924.

4 Sladen J G. Compression sclerotherapy: preparation, technique, complications and results. *Am. J. Surg.*, 1983, **146**, 228-232.

5 Cockett F B. Arterial complications during surgery and sclerotherapy of varicose veins. *Phlebology*, 1986, **1**, 3-6.

6 Batch A J G, Wickremesinghe S S, Gannon M E, Dormandy J A. Randomised trial of bandaging after sclerotherapy for varicose veins. *Br. Med. J.*, 1980, **2**, 423.

7 Reddy P, Wickers J, Terry T, Lamont P, Moller J, Dormandy J. What is the correct period of bandaging following sclerotherapy? *Phlebology*, 1986, **1**, 217-220.

Chapter 4

1 Mullins R J, Lucas C E, Ledgerwood A M. The natural history following venous ligation for civilian injuries. *J. Trauma*, 1980, **20**, 737-743.

2 Timberlake G A, O'Connell R C, Kerstein M D. Venous injury: to repair or to ligate, the dilemma. *J. Vasc. Surg.*, 1986, **4**, 553-558.

3 Rich N M, Hughes C W, Baugh J H. Management of venous injuries. *Ann. Surg.*, 1970, **171**, 218-226.

4 Rich N M, Jarstfer B S, Geer T M. Popliteal artery repair failure: causes and possible prevention. *J. Cardiovasc. Surg.*, 1974, **15**, 340-351.

5 Sullivan W G, Thornton F H, Baker L H, LaPlante E S, Cohen A. Early influence of popliteal vein repair in the treatment of popliteal vessel injuries. *Am. J. Surg.*, 1971, **122**, 528-531.

6 Dale W A, Harris J, Terry R B. Polytetrafluoroethylene reconstruction of the inferior vena cava. *Surgery*, 1984, **95**, 625-630.

7 Smith B M, Mulherin J L, Sawyers J L, Turner B I, Prager R L, Dean R H. Supra vena caval occlusion: principles of operative management. *Ann. Surg.*, 1984, **199**, 656-668.

Chapter 5

1 Haeger K. Complications after outpatient surgery for varicose veins and perforator incompetence. *Vasc. Surg.*, 1970, **4**, 238-243.

2 Nabatoff R A. Complete stripping of varicose veins with the patient on an ambulatory basis. *Am. J. Surg.*, 1972, **124**, 634-637.

3 Richards M T. Ligation and stripping of varicose veins, as an office procedure. *Can. Med. Ass. J.*, 1973, **109**, 215-216.

4 Ruckley C V, Ludgate C M, Maclean M, Espley A J. Major outpatient surgery. *Lancet*, 1973, **ii**, 1193-1196.

5 Ruckley C V, Cuthbertson C, Fenwick N, Prescott R J, Garraway W M. Day care after operations for hernia or varicose veins: a controlled trial. *Br. J. Surg.*, 1978, **65**, 456-459.

6 Garraway W M, Cuthbertson C, Fenwick N, Ruckley C V, Prescott R J. Consumer acceptability of day care after operations for hernia or varicose veins. *J. Epid. & Comm. Health*, 1978, **32**, 219-221.

7 Prescott R J, Cuthbertson C, Fenwick N, Garraway W M, Ruckley C V. Economic aspects of day care after operations for hernia or varicose veins. *J. Epid. & Comm. Health*, 1978, **32**, 222-225.

8 Ruckley C V, Ferguson J B P, Cuthbertson C. Surgical decision making. *Br. J. Surg.*, 1981, **68**, 837-839.

9 Hobson R W, Yeager R A, Lynch T G. Femoral venous trauma: technique for surgical management and early results. *Am. J. Surg.*, 1983, **146**, 220-224.

10 Welch G H, Gilmour D G, Pollock J G. Femoral division during Trendelenburg operation. *J. Roy. Coll. Surg. Edin.*, 1985, **30**, 203-204.

11 Kosinski C. Observations on the superficial venous system of the lower extremities. *J. Anat.*, 1926, **60**, 220-224.

12 Moosman D A, Hartwell S W. The surgical significance of the subfascial course of the lesser saphenous vein. *S,G & O*, 1964, **118**, 761-766.

13 Mercier R. Fouques P, Portal N, Van Neuville G. Anatomie chirurgicale de la veine saphene externe. *J. Chir.*, 1967, **93**, 59-70.

14 Hobbs J T. Errors in the differential diagnosis of incompetence of the popliteal vein and short saphenous vein. *J. Cardiovasc. Surg.*, 1986, **27**, 169-174.

15 Hobbs J T. Per-operative venography to ensure accurate saphenopopliteal ligation. *Br. Med. J.*, 1980, **1**, 1578-1579.

Chapter 6

1 Munn S R, Morton J B, Macbeth W A A G, McLeish A R. To strip or not to strip the long saphenous vein? A varicose veins trial. *Br. J. Surg.*, 1981, **68**, 426-428.

2 Cox S J, Wellwood J M, Martin A. Saphenous nerve injury caused by stripping of the long saphenous vein. *Br. Med. J.*, 1974, **1**, 415-417.

3 Negus D. Should the incompetent saphenous vein be stripped to the ankle? *Phlebology*, 1986, **1**, 33-36.

4 Jacobsen B H, Wallin L. Proximal or distal extraction of the internal saphenous vein? *VASA*, 1975, **4**, 240-242.

5 Rivlin S. The surgical care of primary varicose veins. *Br. J. Surg.*, 1975, **62**, 913-917.

Chapter 8

1 Lofgren E P, Lofgren K A. Recurrence of varicose veins after the stripping operation. *Arch. Surg.*, 1971, **102**, 111-114.

Chapter 9

1 Dodd H, Cockett F B. Varicose veins in pregnancy. In: *The pathology and surgery of the veins of the lower limb.* Churchill Livingstone, London, 1976, Chp.10, 155-158.

2 Rasmussen O O, Jakobsen B H. Post partum persisting pudendal varices—effect of local excision. *Plebology 85.* (Eds) D Negus & G Jantet. Libbey, London, 1986, 229-231.

3 Lechter A, Alvarez A. Pelvic varices and gonadal veins. *Phlebology 85.* (Eds) D Negus & G Jantet. Libbey, London, 1986, 225-228.

Chapter 10

1 Schwartz R S, Osmundson P J, Hollier L. Treatment and prognosis in congenital arteriovenous malformation of the extremity. *Phlebology*, 1986, **1**, 171-180.

2 Klippel M, Trenaunay P. Du naevus varique osteohypertrophique. *Arch. Gen. Med. (Paris)*, 1900, **3**, 641.

Chapter 11

1 Petiti D B, Strom B L, Melmon K L. Duration of warfarin anticoagulant therapy and the probabilities of recurrent thromboembolism and hemorrhage. *Am. J. Med.*, 1986, **81**, 255-259.

2 Coon W W, Coller F A. Some epidemiological considerations of thromboembolism. *S, G & O*, 1959, **109**, 487-501.

3 Morrell T L, Dunnill M S. The post mortem incidence of pulmonary embolism in a hospital population. *Br. J. Surg.*, 1968, **55**, 347-352.

4 MacIntyre I M C, Ruckley C V. Pulmonary embolism—a clinical and autopsy study. *Scot. Med. J.*, 1974, **19**, 20-24.

5 Hull R D, Hirsh J, Carter C J, Jay R M, Dodd P E, Ockelford P A, Coates G, Gill G J, Turpie A G, Doyle D J, Buller H R, Raskob G E. Pulmonary angiography, ventilation lung scanning and venography for clinically suspected pulmonary embolism with abnormal perfusion lung scan. *Ann. Int. Med.*, 1983, **98**, 891-899.

6 Walker M G, Shaw J W, Thomson G J L, Cumming J G R, Lea Thomas M. Subcutaneous calcium heparin versus intravenous sodium heparin in treatment of established acute deep vein thrombosis of the legs: a multicentre prospective randomised trial. *Br. Med. J.*, 1987, **294**, 1189-1192.

7 Verstraete M. New aspects of thrombolysis. *Phlebology 85.* (Eds) D Negus & G Jantet. Libbey, London, 1986, 482-485.

8 Norgren L, Widmer L K. Venous function evaluated by foot volumetry in patients with a previous deep vein thrombosis treated by streptokinase. *VASA*, 1978, **7**, 412-414.

9 Albrechtsson U, Anderson J. Einarsson E, Eklof B, Norgren˙L. Streptokinase treatment of deep venous thrombosis and the post-thrombotic syndrome. *Arch. Surg.*, 1981, **116**, 33-37.

10 Kakkar V V, Paes T R F, Murray W J G. Does thrombolytic therapy prevent the post-phlebitic syndrome? *Phlebology 85.* (Eds) D Negus & G Jantet. Libbey, London, 1986, 481.

11 Roos D B. Congenital anomalies associated with the thoracic outlet syndrome: Anatomy, symptoms, diagnosis and treatment. *Am. J. Surg.*, 1976, **132**, 771-778.

12 De Weese, J A. Management of subclavian obstruction. Chp. 26 in *Surgery of the veins.* (Eds) J J Bergan & J S T Yao. Grune & Stratton, New York, 1985, 365-382.

13 Ruckley C V, Boulton F E, Redhead D. The treatment of venous thrombosis of the upper and lower limbs with 'APSAC' (p-anisoylated streptokinase-plasminogen complex). *Eur. J. Vasc. Surg.*, 1987, **1**, 107-112.

14 Eklof B, Einarsson E, Plate G. Role of thrombectomy and temporary arteriovenous fistula in acute iliofemoral venous thrombosis. Chp. in *Surgery of the veins.* (Eds) J J Bergan & J S T Yao. Grune & Stratton, New York, 1985, 131-144.

15 Gruss Y D. Does surgery have a place in acute venous thrombosis? Chp. in *Vascular surgery issues in current practice.* (Eds) R M Greenhalgh, C W Jamieson & A N Nicolaides. Grune & Stratton, New York, 1986, 395-408.

16 Miles R M, Elsea P W. Clinical evaluation of the serrated vena caval clip. *S, G & O*, 1971, **132**, 581-587.

17 Cimochowski G E, Evans R H, Zarins C K, Lu C T, DeMeester T R. Greenfield filter versus Mobin-Uddin umbrella. *J. Thor. Cardiovasc. Surg.*, 1980, **79**, 358-365.

18 Greenfield L, Peyton R, Crute S, Barnes R. Greenfield caval filter experience. *Arch. Surg.*, 1981, **116**, 1451-1456.

19 Gunther R W, Schild H, Fries A, Storkel S. Vena caval filter to prevent pulmonary embolism: an experimental study. *Radiology*, 1985, **156**, 315-320.

20 Roehm J O F, Gianturco C, Barth M H. Percutaneous interruption of the inferior vena cava: The bird's nest filter. Chp. in *Surgery of the veins*. (Eds) J J Bergen & J S T Yao. Grune & Stratton, New York, 1985, 487-496.

Chapter 12

1 Kleinsasser L J. "Effort" thrombosis of the axillary and subclavian veins: an analysis of sixteen personal cases and fifty-six cases collected from the literature. *Arch. Surg.*, 1949, **59**, 258-265.

2 Swinton N W, Edgett J W, Hall R J. Primary subclavian-axillary vein thrombosis. *Circulation*, 1968, **38**, 737-744.

3 Adams J T, De Weese J A. "Effort" thrombosis of the axillary and subclavian veins. *J. Trauma*, 1971, **11**, 923-928.

4 Tilney N L, Griffiths H J G, Edwards E A. Natural history of major venous thrombosis of the upper extremity. *Arch. Surg.*, 1970, **101**, 792-796.

5 Porter J M, Seaman, A J, Common H H *et al*. Comparison of heparin and streptokinase in the treatment of venous thrombosis. *Am. Surg.*, 1975, **41**, 511-516.

6 Ruckley C V, Boulton F E, Redhead D. Lysis of venous thrombosis with 'APSAC' (p-anisoylated streptokinase-plasminogen complex). *Eur. J. Vasc. Surg.*, 1987, **1**, 107-112.

7 De Weese J A, Adams J T, Gaiser D L. Subclavian venous thrombectomy. *Circulation, 1970,* **41** and **42** (Supp.II), 158-164.

8 Roos D B. Experience with first rib resection for thoracic outlet syndrome. Ann. Surg., 1971, 173, 429-437.

9 De Weese J A. Management of subclavian venous obstruction. Chp. in *Surgery of the veins*. (Eds.) J J Bergen & J S T Yao. Grune & Stratton, New York, 1985, 365-382.

10 Roos D B. Transaxillary approach for first rib resection to relieve thoracic outlet syndrome. *Ann. Surg.*, 1966, **163**, 354-358.

11 Roos D B. Surgical treatment of the thoracic outlet syndromes. Chp. in *Vascular surgery*. (Ed.) C W Jamieson. Baillière Tindall, 1985, 133-146.

Chapter 13

1 Hoare M C, Nicolaides A N, Miles C R, Shull K, Jury R P, Needham T, Dudley H A F. The role of primary varicose veins in venous ulceration. *Surgery*, 1982, **92**, 450-453.

2 Sethia K K, Darke S G. Long saphenous incompetence as a cause of venous ulceration. *Br. J. Surg.*, 1984, **71**, 754-755.

3 Moore D J, Himmel P D, Sumner D S. Distribution of venous valvular incompetence in patients with the post-phlebitic syndrome. *J. Vasc. Surg.*, 1986, **3**, 49-54.

4 Strandness D E, Langlois Y, Cramer M, Thiele B L. Long term sequelae of acute venous thrombosis. *JAMA*, 1983, **250**, 1289-1292.

5 Killewich L A, Martin R, Cramer M, Beach K W, Strandness D E. An objective assessment of the physiologic changes in the post-thrombotic syndrome. *Arch. Surg.*, 1985, **120**, 424-426.

6 Cockett F B, Elgan-Jones D E. The ankle blow-out syndrome. A new approach to the varicose ulcer problem. *Lancet*, 1953, i, 17-23.

7 Linton R R. The post-thrombotic ulceration of the lower extremity: its etiology and surgical treatment. *Ann. Surg.*, 1953, **138**, 415-432.

8 Kistner R L, Sparkhul M D. Surgery in acute and chronic venous disease. *Surgery*, 1979, **85**, 31-43.

9 Kistner R L. In: *Surgery of the veins*. (Eds) J J Bergan & J S T Yao. Grune & Stratton, New York, 1985, Chp. 15, 205-217.

10 Raju S. Venous insufficiency in the lower limb and stasis ulceration. Changing concepts and management. *Ann. Surg.*, 1982, **197**, 221-224.

11 Queral L A, Whitehouse W M, Flinn W R, Neiman H L, Yao J S T, Bergan J J. Surgical correction of chronic deep venous insufficiency by valvular transposition. *Surgery*, 1980, **87**, 688-695.

12 Johnson N D, Queral L A, Flinn W R, Yao J S T, Bergan J J. Late objective assessment of venous valve surgery. *Arch. Surg.*, 1981, **116**, 1461-1466.

13 Taheri S A, Elias S M, Yacobucci G N, Heffner R, Lazae L. Indications and results of vein valve transplant. *J. Cardiovasc. Surg.*, 1986, **27**, 163-167.

14 Palma E C, Esperon R. Vein transplants and grafts in the surgical treatment of the post-phlebitic syndrome. *J. Cardiovasc. Surg.*, 1960, **1**, 94-107.

Chapter 14

1   Bobek K, Cajzl L, Slaisova V, Opatzny K, Barcal R. Etude de la frequence des maladies phlebologiques et de l'influence de quelques facteurs etiologiques. *Phlebologie*, 1966, **19**, 217-230.

2   Widmer L K. *Peripheral venous disorders: prevalence and sociomedical importance.* Hans Huber, Bern, 1978.

3   Dale J J, Callam M J, Ruckley C V, Harper D R, Berrey P N. Chronic ulcers of the leg: a study of prevalence in a Scottish community. *Health Bulletin*, 1983, **41.6**, 310-314.

4   Callam M J, Ruckley C V, Harper D R, Dale J J. Chronic ulceration of the leg: extent of the problem and provision of care. *Br. Med. J.*, 1985, **290**, 1855-1856.

5   Callam M J, Harper D R, Dale J J, Ruckley C V. Chronic ulcer of the leg: clinical history. *Br. Med. J.*, 1987, **1**, 1389-1391.

6   Callam M J, Harper D R, Dale J J, Ruckley C V. Arterial disease in chronic leg ulceration: an underestimated hazard? Lothian and Forth Valley leg ulcer study. *Br. Med. J.*, 1987, **1**, 929-931.

7   Bertelsen S, Gammelgaard A. Surgical treatment of post-thrombotic leg ulcers. *J. Cardiovasc. Surg.*, 1965, **6**, 452-454.

8   Silver D, Gleysteen J J, Rhodes G R. Surgical treatment of the refractory postphlebitic ulcers. *Arch. Surg.*, 1971, **103**, 554-563.

9   Negus D, Friegood A. The effective management of venous ulceration. *Br. J. Surg.*, 1983, **70**, 623-627.

10   Haeger K. Prevention of venous leg ulcer recurrence by a simplified procedure of perforator ligation in ambulant practice. *VASA*, 1984, **13**, 248-250.

11   Deas J, Billings P, Brennan S, Silver I, Leaper D. The toxicity of commonly used antiseptics on fibrolasts in tissue culture. *Phlebology*, 1986, **1**, 205-209.

12   Rundle J S H, Cameron S H, Ruckley C V. New porcine dermis dressing for varicose and traumatic leg ulcers. *Br. Med. J.*, 1976, **1**, 216.

13   Callam M J, Dale J J, Ruckley C V, Harper D R, Prescott R J. A controlled trial of weekly ultrasound therapy in chronic leg ulceration. *Lancet*, 1987, **ii**, 204-205.

14   Burnand K, Clemenson G, Morland M, Jarrett P E M, Browse, N L. Venous lipodermatosclerosis: treatment by fibrinolytic enhancement and elastic compression. *Br. Med. J.*, 1980, **280**, 7-11.

Chapter 16

1   J J Bergan. Conrad Jobst and the development of pressure gradient therapy for venous disease. Chp. in *Surgery of the veins*. (Eds) J J Bergen & J S T Yao. 1985. Grune & Stratton, New York, 529-540.

2   Sigel B, Edestein A L, Felix W R. Compression of the deep venous system of the lower leg during inactive recumbancy. *Arch. Surg.*, 1973, **106**, 38-43.

3   Fentem P H, Goddard M, Gooden B A, Yeung C K. Control of distension of varicose veins achieved by leg bandages, as used after injection sclerotherapy. *Br. Med. J.*, 1976, **2**, 725-727.

4   Horner J, Fernandes e Fernandes J, Nicolaides A N. Value of graduated compression stockings in deep venous insufficiency. *Br. Med. J.*, 1979, **1**, 820-821.

5   Jones N A G, Webb P J, Rees R I, Kakkar V V. A physiological study of elastic compression stockings in venous disorders of the leg. *Br. J. Surg.*, 1980, **67**, 569-572.

6   British Standards Institution report number BS 6612: 1985.

7   Partsch H. Do we need firm compression stockings exerting high pressure? *VASA*, 1984, **13**, 52-57.

8   Chant A D B, Magnussen P, Kershaw C. Support hose and varicose veins. *Br. Med. J.*, 1985, **1**, 204.

9   Raj T B, Goddard M, Makin G S. How long do compression bandages maintain their pressure during ambulatory treatment of varicose veins? *Br. J. Surg.*, 1980, **67**, 122-124.

10   Dale J J, Callam M J, Ruckley C V. How efficient is a compression bandage? *Nursing Times*, 1983, **79**, 49-51.

Index